UNEXPECTED
HEALING

Also by the same author:

BEYOND HEALING
WHERE HAVE YOU GONE, GOD?
LEANING ON A SPIDER'S WEB

UNEXPECTED HEALING

Jennifer Rees Larcombe

Hodder & Stoughton
LONDON SYDNEY AUCKLAND

British Library Cataloguing in Publication Data

Cataloguing in Publication Data
is available from the British Library

ISBN 0-340-55686-2

First published in Great Britain 1991
Fifth impression 1992

Published by Hodder and Stoughton,
a division of Hodder and Stoughton Ltd,
Mill Road, Dunton Green, Sevenoaks, Kent TN13 2YA.
Editorial Office: 47 Bedford Square, London WC1B 3DP.

Photoset by Rowland Phototypesetting Ltd,
Bury St Edmunds, Suffolk

Printed in Great Britain by Clays Ltd, St Ives plc

TO OUR FAMILY DOCTOR

WITH MANY THANKS FOR ALL HIS

KINDNESS, PATIENCE AND CARE

AND

TO ALL 'CARERS'

WHO VOLUNTARILY 'LAY DOWN THEIR OWN
LIVES' FOR DISABLED PEOPLE

PARTICULARLY MY OWN HUSBAND TONY

Foreword

I first met Jenny Rees Larcombe when we recorded a *Highway* programme from Burrswood – a Christian healing centre in Kent.

She had been dependent upon a wheelchair for some years, suffering from chronic encephalitis, and in my interview with her she told me of how she had come to Burrswood hoping for a miracle cure, but it had been denied her. Instead another minor miracle had occurred – she had come to terms with her illness. Her faith was so strong that she could now face up to her disability. There was no bitterness in her and as she spoke quietly and with an almost unbearable serenity, many of those present, including myself and a hard-bitten camera crew were moved to tears. We learned later that she had refused to take her pain-killing drugs that day so that she would be able to talk with a clear mind.

Jenny made a lasting impression on me and caused me to marvel at the way her unquenchable spirit could withstand such severe suffering and still retain her faith. Somehow her example put into perspective all the much lesser trials and tribulations of one's own life.

Imagine my surprise and delight when, some months later, I received a letter from Jenny telling me that her miracle had happened and that she could now walk.

I will not pre-empt what Jenny has to say in the following pages, but the bright-eyed, smiling lady who chatted with me about her wonderful recovery on a subsequent *Highway* from the New Forest was evidence enough for me and for millions of *Highway* viewers, that a remarkable transformation had indeed taken place.

This is a story of courage, of the power of prayer and above all of one woman's refusal to accept defeat.

Harry Secombe

The Story in a Nutshell

In 1982 I developed encephalitis, an inflammation of the brain and meninges which was further complicated by inflamed nerves. The attack nearly proved fatal, and two years later neurological tests showed that it may have left permanent damage. Between 1984 and 1987 I had four more attacks, each of which was as serious, prolonged and life-threatening. Between these acute episodes of illness, the inflammation of the brain, meninges, nerves and muscles seemed to remain in a chronic form and was labelled by the neurologists as Myalgic Encephalomyelitis. These two problems lead to continuous pain, and loss of balance, muscular weakness and fatigue made it necessary for me to use a wheelchair when I needed to walk more than a few yards. Slowness and general lack of coordination, blurred vision and distorted hearing made life as the mother of six children very complicated. Light was painful and my sense of smell and taste were impaired. There was loss of sensation in limbs and also lack of bladder and bowel control.

In November 1984 I was seen by two separate DHSS doctors who sanctioned the spending of thousands of pounds on the adaptation of our house with a lift, automatic door openers, ramps and rails. They also awarded me the mobility allowance, and the attendance allowance, which was later known as the severe disability allowance, at the highest rate. When, two years later, my case was reviewed by the DHSS they said I had deteriorated to the point where regular assessments would no longer be necessary. A polite way of saying they did not expect me to recover. On many occasions, doctors kindly explained that there was no cure for my condition – they could only alleviate the symptoms.

All these things make people feel as if they have joined the ranks of the 'no hopers'. But there is always hope! Something very wonderful happened to me on the afternoon of June 13th 1990. Was it a miracle? To be classed as such by the Medical Bureau at Lourdes, a recovery must be totally impossible medically or by any other natural means – such as the restoration of an amputated leg. Although doctors could offer no cure for my condition, it could have improved (anyway, in part) by itself, just as such conditions as cancer suddenly disappear for no apparent reason. So technically what happened to me was not 'a miracle', yet the Oxford dictionary defines the word as 'a remarkable thing'. My sudden and complete recovery that afternoon was indeed 'a remarkable thing' after eight years of pain and increasing disability. There could be many explanations, and as you read the story I leave you to form your own opinion.

Acknowledgments

THANK YOU TO THE NHS . . .

It is fashionable these days to criticise the National Health Service and devalue the DSS. After eight years of being 'in their power' I have nothing but praise for the universally high standard of care, attention and kindness which I received. In five different hospitals I was seen by countless doctors, nurses, physiotherapists and ancillary helpers. At home I was cared for by our GP, district nurses, occupational therapists and home helps. Although none of these people could make me well again, their professional competence and sheer human kindness helped to make life as a disabled person more than satisfactory. Even the potentially humiliating experience of being assessed for the severe disability allowance, mobility allowance and invalidity benefit was not allowed to rob me of my self-esteem. Only on one isolated occasion, which is amusing in retrospect, was that amazingly high standard of professionalism not maintained. I doubt if anywhere in the world such a record could be equalled.

THANK YOU TO MY FAMILY . . .

My husband Tony and our six children, Sarah, Justyn, Jane, Naomi, Duncan and Richard lived through this story with me and then relived it as they read and discussed the manuscript.

They have kindly allowed me to share many personal things about our lives, our mistakes and our feelings.

THANK YOU TO MY FRIENDS . . .

Carolyn Armitage, editorial director at Hodder and Stoughton, saw this book through several drafts with her usual blend of wisdom and flair. Edward England has also been an invaluable help at every stage. Several people have read the manuscript and given helpful advice: our family doctor, Liz Manning, Stephen Moody and Penny Hill. Other friends have helped in many ways, among them Alison Lewis, Ron and Sue Williams, and Neil and Janet Crisp who lent me their cottage as a refuge in which to write.

THANK YOU TO THE OTHER PEOPLE IN THIS BOOK . . .

This is not only our story, many others were involved over the years and they have kindly allowed me to mention them by name. For some it has required a lot of courage on their part!

MY APOLOGIES . . .

These go to anyone who may have read an earlier book of mine, *Beyond Healing*. You may recognise some of the material at the beginning of this book, but I hope you will find it is presented in a new way and from the standpoint of time.

PART
ONE

Chapter 1

I was wearing an ancient plastic mac, moth-eaten ski pants and wellington boots – standard uniform for a blackberry picker. The ice-cream carton I was clutching was almost full of shiny fat berries and as I wriggled farther into the hedge I was debating whether to make bramble jelly or freeze down a batch of fruit pies. I reached up towards a particularly rich branch of fruit to see a robin inspecting me with his head on one side. The sun felt warm upon my back. Suddenly I experienced one of those moments which come so seldom in a lifetime you wish you could cork them up in a bottle and preserve them for ever. 'I've got everything I ever wanted,' I thought. 'My life is complete.' Happiness sometimes creeps up so gradually over the years it takes you by surprise when you realise it has actually arrived.

Thirty years before, a formidable great-aunt had asked me what I wanted to do in life, thrusting her crumpled face close to mine as she waited for a reply. Backing away from her bristly moustache I said nervously: 'I want to live down a little winding lane in the country, and have lots of children.'

I could imagine it all so clearly – bees humming among the roses, vegetables growing in neat rows and home-made bread ready to come out of the oven. 'I'll have chickens and a goat too so long as it doesn't butt me and . . .' But Auntie, who came from missionary stock, was not impressed.

'That's not a very worthy ambition,' she said disapprovingly.

13

'Well, I'd like to write books,' I ventured, 'and read them aloud to the children after tea.'

Auntie looked at me witheringly through her thick spectacles: 'You'll have to do something about your spelling first.'

I knew my teachers would agree with her, so I kept my dreams safely locked up inside my head where no one could mock them – until I married Tony.

Some people work hard all their lives at turning their dreams into reality. I suppose we were lucky to manage it after only fifteen years of marriage. Anyway, when we arrived in Mayfield we both knew we had found our Utopia. By September 1981 and the day I went blackberry picking we had lived in 'the house down the little winding lane' for six years. The roses, hens and vegetables were just as I had envisaged and I had so many children I was known locally as the Old Woman Who Lived in a Shoe. Only the goat was missing, but we had ducks instead.

With difficulty I extracted myself from the tangled brambles and looked round for the children. In those days I seemed to spend my whole life counting up to six in my head! Jane was still conscientiously filling her tub with blackberries while Duncan with equal concentration filled his mouth. Naomi and Richard had given up altogether and were examining the wonders of an ant-hill. We had left the other two back in the garden.

Over the fields I could see Mayfield – a perfect Sussex village cuddling the top of the hill. From the middle of the clustered roof-tops the church spire pointed up like a finger at the sky.

'This is where I want to be for the rest of my life,' I thought with a sigh of contentment and pictured myself blackberrying with my grandchildren.

> God gives all men all earth to love,
> But, since man's heart is small,
> Ordains for each one spot shall prove
> Belovèd over all.

14

Kipling lived in Sussex too!

'Mum, when's tea time?' asked Duncan. 'You said you'd make scones.' There was never much time for leisurely thoughts in those days!

'Mum!' Our two eldest children were squeezing through the hedge from the garden behind me. 'Can we have tea under the apple tree?' asked Sarah.

'I'm off to find mushrooms,' said Justyn, as he pushed past her.

An hour later we were sitting under the apple tree eating hot scones and home-made bread. All of us, that is, except Justyn and Duncan who were up the tree not under it – they had made sure they took their tea with them. All of them had fair hair and blue eyes. Richard was three, Sarah was thirteen and the others fitted neatly in between.

Tony had been gardening all the afternoon. Now he lay flat on his back on the grass while the children heaped themselves around him. He has always had a 'Pied Piper' quality which causes children to gravitate towards him. At that time he was a teacher adviser based in Tunbridge Wells, ten miles away, but being a father was the first priority in his life. We did everything together and I thought life would always be like that.

Fortunately I managed to preserve the atmosphere of those halcyon days by keeping a diary, though I often wonder how ever I found the time. It became a kind of ritual. First thing in the morning Tony made a pot of tea and I would sit up in bed and record the funny, ordinary bits and pieces of 'yesterday' before they were lost for ever. Looking through the entries for the months which followed I see they were packed with the important events of country life, the autumn flower show, harvest supper, village carnival and the WI Christmas 'do.'

But the following February I describe a nightmare. It woke me up in the dark and I found myself crouching against the wall at the pillow end of the bed. I was shaking all over and my face was wet with tears.

'Tony!' I gasped, but he did not stir. Cautiously I slid out of bed and groped my way down to the kitchen. A nice cup of tea was what I needed. While the kettle boiled I tried to remember the dream, but that was not so easy. I knew I had been standing beside a doctor looking at my family, who seemed to be a vast distance away from me. I was crying and struggling to reach them because they were going through some kind of dreadful experience. The irritating part was that I could not remember any more. So I blamed the cheese on toast I'd had for supper and sat down at the kitchen table to enjoy my tea.

We seemed to do everything round that table: mix the dough, eat our Christmas dinner, play tiddlywinks and struggle with maths homework. It was just the kind of safe world I wanted for my children. 'Good job it was only a dream,' I told myself as I climbed back up to bed.

After dropping Richard off at playgroup the following morning I went for a long walk in the woods. Life with so many energetic children could be quite hectic and I felt I needed to escape sometimes in order to keep my sanity. That was my excuse, but perhaps I just liked walking! It was pouring with rain and very cold, but that did not deter me. I had completely forgotten my dream, and as I set off down the lane I was feeling rather excited. Richard would be starting school later in the year, the last of the brood to leave. After fourteen years of solid motherhood, I would have some free time at last, but what should I do with it? There seemed so many delightful possibilities.

When I finally jumped over the ditch into Fir Toll Wood, however, I felt strangely let down. It had been May when I came here last, and the bluebells and fresh green beech leaves had given the wood a fairyland quality. It was stupid to expect that kind of beauty on a wet day in February, but still the transformation took me by surprise. The winter trees looked bare and stark and the ground which had once been carpeted with flowers was covered with dead brown leaves and ugly fungi. No birds were singing above my head and a nasty, rotting smell hung about the place. As I splashed along by the muddy stream the rain dripped down on my knitted hat until it was soggy. The dark brooding atmosphere of that dream began to come back to me and I suddenly had the oddest thought. My life here in Mayfield was rather like how these woods had been in springtime – packed full of so many lovely things. Would I cope if the 'season' changed and life became dark, bare and wintry – stripped of everything which made it enjoyable?

I sat down suddenly on a damp tree-stump feeling completely out of my depth. This kind of thinking was simply not part of my busy, practical personality and for some reason I felt very frightened. Supposing some disaster really was threatening our lives and no inviting future lay ahead after all?

'I must stop all this morbid nonsense,' I told myself furiously, 'it isn't healthy,' but the feeling of being 'warned' was so vivid I noted it down in my diary.

Probably I would soon have forgotten the whole affair if I had not had rather a strange phone call a few days later.

'Jen?' My friend's voice on the other end of the line sounded unusually diffident, even embarrassed. 'I feel I ought to tell you about a dream I had last night.'

In her dream Tony told her I was dead. I remember sitting down suddenly and feeling as if all the breath had been knocked right out of my body. I had never paid much attention to dreams, but this came too soon after my own to be ignored. If it had been one of my other friends I would probably have laughed and told her she was being ridiculous but she was someone whose judgment and common sense I trusted completely. She certainly believes in dreams and for her they have an uncanny way of coming true.

'Why are you telling me this?' I asked jerkily.

'Perhaps you need to prepare yourself?' she replied gently.

The following Sunday I remember looking round at the family during lunch. The boys sat at one side of the kitchen table, the girls on the other and Tony down at the far end.

17

They were all laughing loudly at some joke and were blissfully unaware of the ice-cold fear that had been attacking me since I spoke to my friend. That morning we had all sat in the same pew in church and in the afternoon we would probably go on a long muddy walk and come home to toast crumpets by the fire. It seemed outrageous that this safe, happy life we had so carefully constructed should ever be destroyed. Surely I was imagining these silly forebodings?

'I'm going to start the spring-cleaning this week,' I announced brightly. Everyone groaned, but I felt that vigorous activity might restore my equilibrium. During the next few days I battered the house into submission and ate a shameful quantity of chocolate biscuits, but nothing would shake off that fear.

I wanted to discuss it all with Tony. We never kept anything from each other, but it seemed rather mean to worry him over something which was probably only a mixture of coincidence and my vivid imagination.

It was late one evening the following week when I finally allowed myself to stop and think. Tony was attending a maths conference, the children were in bed and, apart from a hefty pile of mending, I could not find anything else to occupy my mind.

'This is stupid!' I said suddenly and dropped the sock I was darning. I was young, strong and extremely happy. The possibility that I might die one day had never really occurred to me before. I felt terribly alone sitting there. I longed to talk to someone, but death was a subject I felt I could not discuss, not even with the friend who had so recently rung me.

'Oh God, don't let me have to die,' I whispered. 'I'm only thirty-nine and life's such fun.' I had never been very good at praying, and the arrival of so many children had reduced me to communicating with the Almighty while I cleaned the bath or had my hands in the greasy sink. That night, however, I felt the seriousness of the occasion demanded a certain formality. So I pushed the piles of mending out of the way and knelt on the floor by the sofa. The lamplight and the flickering fire were so comforting that at last I was able to explore my fear from every angle. Actually, I soon discovered that being dead did not worry me. My Christian faith assured me it would only be a beginning, but heaven did not appeal to me much; I had already created a perfectly satisfactory one down here in Mayfield. The actual moment of death was what I really feared most. What would it feel like? Would it be painful? Then I suddenly thought about Jane.

Only five of the children were ours by birth. Jane had not come to us until she was seven. Her parents were our friends, but when Jane was only three her mother died of cancer, and four years later her father had a massive heart attack. Jane found him lying on the landing outside her bedroom in the middle of the night. She had always been terrified of the dark, but she ran up and down the road in her bare feet, trying to find someone who would help. She had to knock on every door before a light finally came on. When the social worker brought her to our house at teatime the following day she still had no idea her father was dead. It was Naomi's sixth birthday party and we were shovelling the jelly and crisps from the floor when they arrived. Tony took her away from the balloons and the festivities and sat her down under the apple tree.

'That's all right,' she said when he finished his unenviable task. 'I'll stay here with you instead. Can I go on the swing now, please?' Perhaps her father had sensed this might happen, because his will made it clear he wanted us to be her guardians. A litter of orphaned kittens and her absorbing interest in Richard, who was then only a baby, had helped her initially, but she was so shattered by her double bereavement that it took the combined efforts of the whole family to mend her over the next few years. It was hardly surprising that illness of any kind terrified her – I only had to sneeze for her to clutch my jumper with both hands and cling on tight for the rest of the day.

'You won't die will you?' she used to say frequently. To which I always replied: 'Of course not, I'm as strong as a horse. I promise I'll live to a hundred.'

She would always relax then – she trusted me completely. 'I've got to survive even if it's only for her sake,' I told myself firmly. I stood up stiffly from my unaccustomed position and began to feel better.

Even my sense of humour seemed to return as I looked at the pile of badly darned socks. I loathed mending, and if I was safely out of the way Tony could marry someone who was rather better at the job. I ran through a mental list of my eligible friends and discovered an excellent female to fill the the vacancy, but as I imagined her clucking nervously at my six noisy children I began to laugh out loud. No! I wasn't going to die and leave everything I loved to someone like her. These premonitions were absurd. Trouble was something which happened to other people – not to us. I threw the mending back into the sewing drawer and went up to bed.

Apart from describing those events in my diary I don't think I gave them another thought. Life went flowing happily on through Easter and the explosion of a new spring. Yet certain phrases begin to crop up sometimes on the pages rather like little wispy clouds in a blue sky.

'Can't seem to get over this silly flu.'

'Feel tired all the time these days.'

'My legs and arms seem like heavy tubes of wet sand.'

All these symptoms were so vague I never dreamt of admitting how I felt anywhere else except my diary. Yet the sore throat persisted for three months and the headache simply would not go away. Tony and I seemed to live by the theory that if you ignored illness, eventually it just went away. The body heals itself. It worked well enough, simply because as a family we were all so healthy.

By the beginning of May the 'wisps' in my diary had formed themselves into a bank of black storm clouds.

'What's the matter with me?' I kept asking as the pain in my head began to spread down my neck and spine. I had always had a stupid guilt feeling about being ill. Somehow it felt like failure to me. 'I ought to be one hundred per cent fit, with a healthy life-style like mine,' I thought, as I swallowed vitamin pills like sweets and took myself on long route-marches along the muddy bridle paths. Often I walked with a friend who was a great fitness fanatic.

'It's mind over matter,' she would tell me enthusiastically. 'You don't have to be ill if you don't want to be – think healthy. People who are unhappy or over-stretched use illness as a way of escape.' Her words did nothing for my self-condemnation!

'May 16th, 1982. Bluebell picnic in Fir Toll Wood.' Everything was beautiful there once again, but I remember flopping down against a tree-trunk and shutting my aching eyes.

'Come and paddle in the stream, Mum,' called Richard. 'Naomi keeps turning over stones and showing me little wiggling things.'

'Mayfly larvae,' I mumbled without opening my eyes. 'Go and see if you can find any more.' The pungent scent of the bluebells seemed to rise thick and warm from the earth beneath me but all I wanted to do was crawl into my bed in a dark room and sleep for days.

'Mummy, what *is* the matter?' asked Naomi. Even at ten she had a great capacity for sensing other people's feelings.

'I'm fine,' I said hastily, opening my eyes, but perhaps that was the day I first realised that I was not.

Tony must have seen I was far from well that spring but I would never have admitted to him how I really felt. When I began falling over because I was so giddy the children thought it was a huge joke.

'Don't tell Daddy about this,' I warned them when I struggled to my feet for the third time in one afternoon. I made a supreme effort to be brisk and cheerful because I was so afraid he might cart me straight off to the doctor. That would have seemed like a final defeat. I was safe while I could still control the situation by denying that it was real.

Like many other mothers, I did not want to think the family could do without me, even for a day. To be in charge of my environment mattered to me intensely. So I used to crawl back into bed while the children were at school or playgroup and then drag myself up in time to meet them again.

On May 27th I was trying to clean the bath. The pain in my head was severe by then, and my neck was completely stiff. I could not allow myself to think of the implications, so I riveted all my attention on the dirty tidemark instead. 'Just concentrate on this little job and then the next one,' I kept telling myself firmly.

Suddenly I panicked. I was so giddy my brain seemed to be swirling round inside my skull at an alarming rate. I could not make my arm bend or my hand grip the sponge – my whole body felt distant and unreal.

'This is what it feels like to go mad!' I gasped as I tried to focus my eyes on the taps. I could see four – not two. It was the first time I had felt trapped inside a body which was out of my control. It felt as terrifying as hurtling down a steep hill inside a car without brakes or a steering-wheel.

That last evening at home was not a pleasant one. I knew by then that the doctor was coming in the morning. Every time I tried to get up and go downstairs my legs buckled underneath me. All I could do was lie there and listen to the chaos below. Tony had the vegetable garden to water, so Sarah was obviously taking charge of supper and the boys were definitely not making her job an easy one. Every time I closed my eyes I felt someone was watching me, and Jane's reproachful face would be peeping round my bedroom door. Somehow I could not find any words to reassure her this time.

When Sarah marched Duncan and Richard off for a bath, the proceedings sounded more like a water polo match and I cringed as I thought of the ceiling below. Justyn 'kindly' turned the television up extra loud because he thought I would not want to miss the latest news of the Falklands War, and Naomi dropped a tray of crockery. In desperation I pulled the duvet up over my head. 'I wish I could go somewhere safe, a long way away, and stay there for a considerable length of time,' I thought. And my wish was granted.

Chapter 2

Of course it wasn't really happening to me. I was completely detached from the woman who lay in the back of the ambulance. I did not even mind that it was a stranger in uniform who sat beside me and not Tony – Richard needed him far more than I did. All I wanted to do was to sleep. Vaguely I remembered the doctor's visit earlier that morning. He had only needed to make a brief examination before he hurried downstairs to ring for the ambulance.

When we arrived in the Emergency Department of the Kent and Sussex Hospital I felt quite at home. I had spent many hours there in the past. Our children have always been the kind who fall out of trees and break their arms or cut themselves open on barbed-wire fences. But there was no waiting in long queues for me that day, my trolley was swirled through the double doors at high speed and someone shouted:

'Ah, the encephalitis, put it straight in there.'

People swarmed round me, but they were all upside down from my position – their mouths were where their eyes should be. I discovered I was able to escape from them all simply by sliding under a warm woolly blanket of sleep. Its drowsy folds became more real to me than the disturbing things which were happening in the bustling world around me. Now and again my 'blanket' was wrenched away by voices which asked me questions or hands which held sharp needles but most of the time I slept.

Only when one particular pair of grey eyes appeared above me did I make an effort to concentrate. They belonged to a young doctor with untidy fair hair and the nicest smile I have ever met. He actually took the trouble to explain everything he intended to do, before he did it.

'I'm just going to stick this needle into your spine to draw off some of the fluid for testing.' He could even make a lumbar puncture sound like a treat!

'What's the matter with me?' I managed to ask him at some point during the day. I remember wondering why all my words ran into one another so strangely and I hoped this nice young man would not think I was a junkie. He came to sit down next to the bed so his face was on a level with mine and he said:

'I think you have encephalitis* and I suspect the lining of your heart is also inflamed. Does all that worry you?' It should have done because I had contracted encephalitis before we were married, and it had taken me more than two years to recover from its effects. But his words meant no more to me than if he had told me I had a cold in the head. He was treating me as if I was still a person and that was all that mattered just then.

It was the glare of the searchlights on the ceiling which next woke me. Probably the lighting was quite subdued but my eyes had become ultrasensitive.

'When's it going to be night?' I whispered to a nurse in desperation.

'It's night-time now,' she replied kindly, 'but the people in this ward are so ill we have to keep the lights on all the time.'

'Poor things,' I remember thinking, 'but I wonder what I'm doing in here with them.' When she covered my eyes with a cold damp flannel, I was so grateful I only wished I could remember the right way of saying 'thank you'.

---

* Encephalitis is an acute inflammation of the brain and meninges (the membranes that surround the brain), usually caused by a viral infection. In most cases encephalitis is a serious and life-threatening condition. Also in most cases there is no known effective treatment. Depending on the cause of the encephalitis some patients die, some are left with brain damage and others make a complete recovery.

It was not only light which bothered me. Sound was also magnified and distorted alarmingly. An ordinary remark felt as if it was being yelled at me through a megaphone and if someone touched the bed I became so dizzy I felt as if I was spinning off into outer space. By then the pain in my head was so bad I remember biting the inside of my cheeks until they were raw and lumpy.

'We're going to put you out of your misery, Mrs Larcombe.' It was the owner of the grey eyes and he had yet another needle in his hand. 'This is heroin – diamorphine,' he added.

'He really does think I'm a junkie,' I thought, but I was a long way past caring.

I cannot remember anything very much for at least a week after that, except for the ducks and geese which I was convinced they kept piling on top of my bed! I told myself the only reason I could not move my legs was because a large goat was sitting on top of them. Apparently they put me into a small room off the ward where I would be away from noise and movement and could be nursed in semi-darkness. They also put cot sides up around me because of convulsions, but at the time I thought it was a sensible way of penning the goat!

I remember someone trying to help me sip tea through the plastic spout of a feeding cup and feeling furious when I could not remember how to swallow. It also seemed very strange when people kept on shining a torch in my eyes while they asked my name and what day it was. Why wake someone from a lovely sleep I wondered, simply for information they must have known anyway!

Often I used to open my eyes and find the hospital chaplain, George Swannell, sitting silently by my bed. Although I had no sensation in my limbs, I always knew when he was holding my hand. In that crazy, painful world which separated me from everything familiar, touch became tremendously important. People seemed to be able to transmit their love and strength best through their hands. At that stage I was

25

really too ill to miss the children, but I ached for Tony. He was trying so hard to keep the familiar routine going at home for their sakes, so he could only slip in to see me at odd moments. I always seemed to be asleep when he did manage to come, so I thought he had abandoned me. At home we were hardly ever apart, so being separated like this was the hardest thing of all for both of us. Tony felt torn in half, knowing he was needed in two places at once.

One day I became aware of a great deal of noise round my cot. A large crowd of people seemed to be filling the room and discussing me as if I was not there. 'They think I can't hear them,' I thought, feeling slightly amused. They were talking about my doubtful future with such brutal frankness that I wondered whatever made them think I was *that* ill!

One of them seemed much bigger than the rest and infinitely more important – he was not wearing a white coat. As he towered over me he kept tapping the side of the bed with his knee. The effect of the slight movement was catastrophic and I wanted to scream at him to go away and leave me in peace, but no sound would come out of my mouth. He continued to stand looking solemnly down at me while I struggled desperately to remember how to speak. Finally I managed the word, 'Stop.' It came out rather like a rusty squeak, but he looked inordinately pleased and stopped at once.

'We're going to have to send you to London tomorrow, Mrs Larcombe.' I wondered why he needed to shout so loudly. Did he think I was deaf? 'They have better equipment up there.' I hated the thought of moving at all. Being turned by two nurses every few hours was bad enough. I wondered if he would expect me to go by myself on the train. However would I manage the goat and all those geese on the underground? My mind still seemed unable to admit that anything was wrong with my body. I was convinced that I was quite capable of getting up and walking about if I chose to exert myself sufficiently. Perhaps it was simply a strategy for coping with my fear.

After some final deafening orders to Sister they all stamped loudly out of the room and I sighed with relief.

Later that day, I heard the words, 'condition worsening', and I finally began to appreciate that something was going wrong with my body. Gradually I seemed to be drifting farther away from reality, like a rowing boat without oars, being pulled out to sea by a strong current. There seemed to be a great increase in the activity around my bed and most of the time Sister herself looked after me personally. I felt honoured and the drifting sensation was rather pleasant until I suddenly heard the voice of the ward domestic outside the door.

'Don't mop in there today, June, that one's dying.'

'No I'm not,' I thought indignantly, 'or am I?'

It is a terrible feeling to panic violently and yet not be able to express your feelings in any way. I wanted to flail my arms, kick my legs and scream for help at the top of my voice, but I could do nothing but lie there looking as if I was asleep. I could not even allow myself to escape into the delicious drowsiness any more; I was afraid that if I went to sleep I might never wake up again.

Then at last Tony was there. I could see his face quite clearly spliced into two by the horizontal cot bars and yet I could not reach out my hands to touch him. I wondered why he looked so ill in the gloomy half-light and why he just sat there – not saying anything at all. If I were dying then I needed to tell him all kinds of things which at the time seemed vitally important. I wanted to say, 'Don't forget Jane only likes peanut butter in her school lunch-box, and Naomi can't stand it.'

Suddenly I was angry. Not with the illness or the doctors who could not cure it, but irrationally angry with Tony himself. In fact I wanted to bite him – hard! He ought to be able to do something to stop this powerful force which was wrenching us apart and ruining everything. He could mend the chicken house roof, unblock the drains, soothe a frightened child – in fact he always managed to solve every family crisis that came along. So why not this one? I sensed he was angry, too, perhaps for exactly the same reason. The rage neither of us could express separated us more completely than the metal cot bars, and when I next opened my eyes he had gone. I will never forget the desolation of that moment and I knew there was something vital I had failed to tell him. He must not feel bad about marrying again. He would need someone to care for him and be a mother to the children. I was wondering miserably how I could manage to communicate that message to him when a nurse called Rhoda came in to see me. It was easier to speak to her, perhaps because I felt more detached and I managed to gather enough energy to dictate a short note. The hospital chaplain promised to deliver it to Tony . . . afterwards. I felt quite exhausted with the effort but very much more peaceful.

During the evening, Sister lent over me and whispered, 'Someone's here to see you – the minister of your church.' She looked as if she thought he had come to give me the last rites but, as Brian and his wife Penny crept into the room, a feeling of unutterable relief spread over me. They had been on holiday since the day I left home in the ambulance, and I knew I had been holding on – just waiting for them to come. Now I felt safe – everything would be all right – the fear and the struggling were over.

They sat down by my cot and gripped my hands through the bars. Again I wanted to say so much, but I only managed to mumble something inane about going to heaven.

'We know,' said Brian in a strangely jerky voice – quite unlike his own. 'But I'm going to pray for you anyway, Jen, and then we'll see what happens.'

As I closed my eyes, the sound of his rich velvety voice began to fade away. Remembering to breathe was too much of an effort, and I realised that it was far easier just not to bother. The discovery made me feel quite emancipated. At the end of the bed, just over my left foot I could see a gentle light beginning to glow. Gradually it grew brighter. 'That's curious,' I thought. Light of any kind had been painful for so long, yet here was a brightness which did not hurt my eyes; in fact it felt oddly inviting. A cave seemed to be opening up in the darkness of the wall by the wash basin, leading up and out of the room. I found I was floating effortlessly away from the body which lay on the bed. Moving my arms and legs was no longer painful and I could even turn somersaults. It was rather like free falling from an aircraft, except that I was going up and not down. 'So this is what dying feels like,' I thought. 'If I had known it was like this I wouldn't have worried, and at the far end of this tunnel I'm actually going to meet God, at long last.'

The thought was not frightening at all. I had wanted to know what God was really like ever since I was three. As a child I was terrified of the dark and I had woken one night too afraid to move. Inside my head I remember calling out to God and feeling sure he would do something to help me. Instantly a bird began to sing outside the thick bedroom curtains and another answered it. Soon it sounded as if every bird in the wood must have flown into our garden and was singing outside my window. I had never heard of the dawn chorus, so I thought the whole thing had been arranged by God just for my benefit! As I grew up I soon realised I was wrong, but I never lost the conviction that God was on my side. Now at last I was going to see Him and the thought was most exciting.

But I didn't meet God after all, and I have often wondered if Brian's prayers had anything to do with that. I knew I was standing on the threshold of somewhere infinitely beautiful and behind and below me was the darkness and pain I had left behind. The familiar presence I had known since childhood seemed to be waiting for me, but I saw nothing except light. Thousands of different shades of coloured light. It was quite indescribably lovely. I wanted to press on eagerly into the place which made my own familiar world at home seem like a poor counterfeit, but something seemed to be stopping me. I knew that down in the darkness below were Tony and the children. I pictured them huddled into a pathetic little group. Somehow I realised I was being given a choice. I could go back to them, or on into all the beauty and freedom which lay ahead. I felt disconcerted. I hate making decisions at the best of times.

'I'm too tired to choose,' I thought fretfully, but everything seemed to be waiting for me to do so. It was with a strange feeling of disappointment that I decided to go back to my family. Then I seemed to hear these words:

'From this moment you will begin to recover and go back. It is going to be a struggle, but I will give you my strength.'

The pain was waiting to trap me as I felt the body on the bed closing round me once again. Brian was still praying but he finished rapidly as nurses buzzed round the bed. I think I managed to mutter something about being better before he and Penny disappeared from view.

The night which followed felt interminable. The sense of anticlimax was devastating as I lay in the dark remembering all those glorious colours. My condition was definitely much improved; I could even talk to the night staff, but I discovered that being better meant I could no longer escape under that blanket of sleepy unconsciousness. I was wide awake and starkly aware of my surroundings for the first time since I left home. The goats and the geese were gone for good, so there was obviously some other more sinister reason why my legs were so difficult to move. There was also the horrid thought that in the morning I would have to go to London. Yes, definitely I should never have come back to a miserable world like this when being dead was obviously such a happy state to be in.

A few days later when Rhoda came to see me again, she helped me to record the whole experience in detail while it was all fresh in my mind. I actually thought I had gone through something unique, as once I had imagined the dawn chorus was just for me. It was not until I later published an account of the events of June 2nd, 1982 that

I realised the 'near death experience,' as it is called, is very common indeed (and much research has already been done into it). People wrote to me describing their own 'near misses' and I was even summoned to the BBC who were making a programme on the subject. In the studio, Tony and I were introduced to a man who had spent years talking to newly resuscitated patients and he had published a fat book on his findings.

'All that you describe is very common,' he said enthusiastically. 'In fact you are a textbook case.' Feeling slightly flattened, I asked him:

'Is it always lovely to die then?' Glancing at our producer he lowered his voice and said, 'I won't say this on the programme for obvious reasons, but sometimes it can be very unpleasant indeed. The patient feels he is being pulled downwards into darkness and becomes extremely afraid. People who have that kind of experience seem to suppress the memory of it very quickly. You couldn't live, could you,' he added with a shrug, 'if you knew death was going to be like that?' I said I supposed you couldn't – after all he was the expert.

While I was lying awake all through that long night, Tony could not sleep either. He thinks he spent most of the time prowling around the house, waiting for the phone to ring. While it was still dark, and long before the children were awake, he dressed, jumped in the car and drove the ten miles to the hospital. He did not really expect I would still be there when he peeped through the round glass porthole in the door of my room. When I saw him I cried with relief – and so did he. I felt so much better than I had done the previous day, we were even able to talk.

'I don't want to go to London,' I told him. 'I'll never cope with all the noise and light.' He fumbled in his pockets and produced his own pair of extra dark sunglasses and closed my fingers round them.

'They'll help a lot,' he said as he dashed away to wake the children. Those glasses were very special to me because they were something of him which I could take with me. We both knew he would not be able to come up and see me very often in London, but I was alive and one day I would go home to him again. That was all that mattered.

Chapter 3

The journey to London was rather pleasant in the end, and I definitely did not have to go on the train. In fact I remember being told the ambulance was one of the best in the country, extra smooth and containing all the most modern equipment. Sister packed my ears with cotton wool to deaden the sound, fixed Tony's dark glasses on my nose and after her parting shot – with the needle – I knew little during the ride. All I remember is the straw yellow hair of my accompanying nurse. She looked just like Jane's favourite doll.

When I finally struggled out of my drugged sleep I discovered the bustling, high pressure world of a large teaching hospital was very different from my quiet little room in the Kent and Sussex. It was one of the best neurological departments in the land, run by a brilliant sister, but even the finest ward can have its staffing emergency. It was just unlucky for me that I happened to arrive when Sister was away on leave.

'Open your eyes, Mrs Larcombe, come on, open your eyes at once!' The rasping voice grated on me badly. Piercing white sunlight seemed to attack me from every angle. I was lying in a glass cubicle which had windows on all sides.

'This is Bright Ward,' announced the voice, and I could not help thinking it was aptly named.

'Oh please close the curtains,' I mumbled.

'No,' was the abrupt reply. 'I have a great many notes to make and I can't write in the dark.' I thanked God for Tony's dark glasses and gritted my teeth. 'Come along now, Mrs Larcombe, wake up, we've got work to do.' She was a young house physician, new to her job, and she had probably been on duty without sleep for far too many hours. However many times I told myself all that, she still reminded me of a Nazi guard in a film I had once seen.

The cross-examination seemed to go on interminably, while fatigue like a thick black hood kept on slipping down over my head.

'It's no wonder you can't hear me,' she shouted when she discovered Sister's cotton wool and, pulling it from my ears, she dropped it on the floor. 'Now how many children have you? And what are their dates of birth?' I simply could not remember and I began to feel like a pulverised idiot. In fact I have had nightmares about her ever since. I hear her voice coming up the corridor towards me and I cringe under the bedclothes. Perhaps she had been taught that kind of technique to rouse semi-comatose patients from their torpor, but she frightened me back into mine. When she discovered the plaster the doctor with the nice grey eyes had stuck on my back after the lumber puncture she snorted with disgust and ripped it off without warning. Perhaps she was simply testing to see how much sensation I still had left, and for once I was glad I had practically none.

'What kind of an idiot put all this stuff on?' she snapped. 'Really! These provincial hospitals!' It must have been about then that she fell over my catheter bag and swore dreadfully. 'I can't see if you're looking at me when you're wearing those ridiculous sunglasses.' When she snatched them away I felt she had severed me from Tony, and all my security was lost.

If I had not been so ill I would probably have been rude back or even managed to make her laugh, but when you are very weak unkindness, however unintentional, frightens you badly.

'Whatever have I done wrong?' I kept wondering. 'Why is she so cross with me?' If she had been one of those glamorous young doctors in TV hospital dramas, her bad mood would all be explained by a terrible row with her boyfriend. Perhaps that kind of thing happens in real life too, I kept on telling myself. But it was not so easy to keep on making excuses for her later in the week. I frequently heard her bullying and shouting at other patients, some of whom were elderly, confused, or who possessed very little English. How very different she was from her counterpart with the grey eyes.

Since meeting her I have encountered scores of NHS doctors and nurses, in five different hospitals. She was the one isolated exception to a remarkably high standard of kindness and care, but I could certainly have done without her particular bedside manner that day.

The phone in Sister's office next door rang loudly and, when she went off to answer it, I sighed with relief and groped guiltily for Tony's sunglasses. I thought she had gone but almost at once she pounced back at me through the door.

'They're ready for you down in the EEG department, so we're sending you right down for the electroencephalogram. After that you'll go straight on for a brain scan and then X-rays.'

'Please,' I begged timidly, 'could I have a drink of water first?' My throat felt parched and raw with thirst after not being able to swallow for so long. She glanced at the locker.

'They haven't been round with the water jugs yet,' she said. 'They're very short-staffed. You'll just have to wait, we can't keep the technicians hanging round.'

To my horror I saw a wheelchair approaching my bed. I had been lying completely flat for more than a week. Suddenly to be forced upright was terrifying. Even a few minutes in a comfortable armchair would have been traumatic at first. Someone heaved me into the wheelchair as if I were a sack of potatoes, and because there was no neck support my head lolled about like a rag doll – short of stuffing.

'I must lie down,' I gasped in terror as the room began to spin round me.

'Trolleys take two porters,' she snapped, 'and they're frantically busy today. This nurse will go with you, so you'll be all right.' The male nurse looked distinctly cross.

As the wheelchair moved off along the corridor I

experienced the most ghastly moments of my life. The vertigo from which I was suffering made me feel we were travelling at high speed, zooming round corners and plunging down into deep valleys. Sometimes we even seemed to be racing upside down along the ceiling like a speeded up version of the worst kind of fairground ride. My head flopped about, increasing the pain in my neck to an alarming level. Someone was making a very strange noise. It echoed about the bare corridor and reminded me of a terrified animal caught in a trap.

'Fancy anyone letting themselves behave like that,' I thought, remembering how I had proudly managed to give birth to all my babies without resorting to gas and air. When I gradually realised the appalling sounds were coming from me, I felt publicly shamed. I struggled to get my hand up high enough to ram it into my mouth like a gag, but the effort was too much for me.

Behind me the nurse and the porter chatted together and cracked jokes. Perhaps transporting noisy lunatics was an everyday occurrence for them.

Suddenly we were approaching what appeared to be a solid wall at high speed. I wanted to shout, 'Look out' but I seemed to have run right out of breath. Actually we were only going through a set of double Perspex doors and the wheels of the chair forced them apart easily, but to me it felt as if we must crash head on. The porter behind me was whistling as he shot the chair over some bumps and swerved violently to avoid a trolley.

I began to gasp for breath wildly and just when I simply could not take any more, a strange thing happened. I had wanted to meet God the night before and had failed to do so, but suddenly I felt Christ himself was right there in that concrete corridor, experiencing the pain, fear and humiliation with me. He knew from experience what it was like. He seemed to care what happened to me in this lowest moment of my life, even if no one else did. For some reason I felt completely safe again and even though I knew I was fainting it did not matter any more. Just before I slid forward on to the ground, dragging all my tubes with me, I remember asking him not to let me lose Tony's sunglasses.

'A patient in this condition should never have been in a wheelchair; fetch a trolley at once,' boomed a voice of authority as I struggled out of the swirling blackness. Cautiously I opened my eyes only to be confronted by a positive jungle of legs. Voices barked orders and hands poked an oxygen mask, stethoscope and yet another needle in my direction. Tony's glasses were no longer on my nose so I hurriedly closed my eyes again and hoped one of the many feet would not step on them.

By the time I arrived back in the ward, thirst had become an obsession. There, far above my head, on top of the high locker stood a jug of water. It haunted me like a mirage as I lay there helplessly looking at it. Perhaps it might help to suck my flannel, but then I noticed all my possessions were still in the grey polythene bag on the far side of the room. No one had yet had time to unpack it for me. If they had only put it within my reach I might not have experienced such a terrible feeling of loss at being severed from everything safe and familiar. But perhaps I only felt like that because Tony's glasses were gone.

I could have rung for a nurse, but the bell was hanging out of reach behind the back of the bed. Even if I had found it I doubt if I would have dared. All the staff looked like frenzied lemmings, scurrying up and down the corridor – and very fierce lemmings at that!

Then I noticed something. In a little slot at the side of the locker was a small book. My fingers did not really seem to be part of me any more, but with a great deal of concentration I managed to slide it on to the bed. It was one of those tiny Gideon Testaments which always seem to turn up in hotels and hospitals. Of course my vision was much too blurred to make reading possible, but as I lay with it open on my tummy I felt it connected me with home and that was very comforting. A drug trolley was bound to come round eventually, I told myself, and they always gave you water to swallow your pills. I might even dare to ask them to pull the curtains and to find Tony's photograph from my bag. I lay there straining my ears for the rumble of its wheels. The pain was unbearable again, but it was not as bad as the thirst. At last I heard the trolley coming up the corridor between the rows of glass cubicles. It was only a matter of time now. It stopped at last right outside my door and two faces peered in at me.

'Look, she's reading,' said one to the other, 'she wouldn't be doing that if she was in pain,' and before I could remember how to shout they were gone.

The next day could not have been more different, even if it did start in rather an unusual way. I was woken while it was still almost dark by a man dancing round my bed. He was stark naked. That was my initiation into the doubtful advantages of a mixed ward. He was hustled away by two sweating night nurses, one of whom came back later to explain he was 'a brain tumour'. He looked more like a ballet dancer to me.

At eight o'clock something magical happened. Sister came back from her holiday. Within minutes she had restored the ward to a state of purring efficiency and suddenly all the scowling lemmings of yesterday turned out to be human after all. In fact several of them became special friends and the cross-looking male nurse even brought his wife and baby to wave at me through the window on his day off. The high spot of the day was reached when the 'whistling porter' padded into my room with Tony's sunglasses in his hand.

'Found them under the radiator,' he said, and actually smiled. I was so pleased I managed to swallow some brown bread and butter and felt as if I had been to the Lord Mayor's banquet.

Chapter 4

Bright Ward was a different place after that and I became very fond of my small glass world. All the same it was rather boring lying flat all day long so I was delighted when the consultant finally said, 'I think you're ready to leave us now.' I thought he meant I could go home.

'That *is* good!' I said happily. 'My family are missing me so much.'

'Yes, they'll be able to come and visit you much more easily in the Kent and Sussex,' he added, and I felt my smile beginning to slip.

'But why have I got to go back there?' I asked tensely.

'Well, your brain scan showed some disturbance, and while we have to hope that will not be of a lasting nature, you have been extremely ill. I'm afraid it will take you a very long time before you could possibly be fit enough to go home to all those children.' I felt stunned. I had known people in the village go into hospital for horrendous operations and be back ten days later, eager to dig their potatoes.

'There must be something you can do,' I insisted.

'I'm afraid rest is all we can offer you,' he said quietly. 'Good luck.'

'Rest!' I thought indignantly as he walked away down the corridor with his terrifying assistant stalking along behind him. I loathe the word rest and I am only truly relaxed when I am doing ten things at once and at high speed. Sitting still makes me fidgety.

Perhaps that was the reason why I enjoyed life more than

I could have expected in the large general ward when I was once again deposited in the Kent and Sussex. Even though I could not be part of the constant activity there was always something interesting to watch – and laugh at too. I was even allowed to be propped up on pillows which gave me a better view.

When you have nothing else to do all day but watch other human beings it is surprising how well you get to know them. Although I never spoke to the old lady in the bed across the ward, I would certainly include her among the most special people I have ever encountered. Mrs Pennington sparkled at everyone who came near her bed. Even though she must have been ninety, the staff all adored her. However ill she had been all day, the moment her elderly husband came shuffling up the ward at visiting time, she seemed to discover enough energy to flirt with him like a chirpy little sparrow.

'I'm so much better, dear,' she would shout into his hearing aid, 'I'll be home any day now to look after you.' You obviously don't have to be young to be in love, but as soon as he had gone she would collapse into her pillows, so exhausted the nurses always put an oxygen mask over her face to revive her. In spite of our communication problem we became very good friends. She would send her husband across with little messages and I would send her back my grapes – pretending I did not like them. I used to love watching the devoted way the old man peeled and stoned them for her with his shaky old hands.

'If I ever manage to write a novel,' I thought, 'I'll use her as the main character.' And I whiled away many a dull hour making up stories about her romantic past.

The morning she died was terrible. We were all having breakfast at eight o'clock and she smiled across at me as usual and waved her slice of brown bread. The next time I looked up there were curtains round her bed and Sister was running to the telephone. The frenzied activity had ceased by the time I was wheeled back from the bathroom. Soon we all had curtains drawn round our beds, and through the gap in mine

I saw two porters pushing away a long metal box on wheels.

By lunch-time a new lady was eating roast beef in Mrs Pennington's bed. No gentle old man came shuffling in at three o'clock that day with a clean nightie and a bottle of milk stout. With my own experience of death so fresh in my mind, I had to feel pleased for Mrs Pennington, but however beautiful death may be for the person who is dying it is ugly and brutally final for the people left behind. So I cried when I thought of that lonely old man and the ward felt bleak and lonely without Mrs Pennington's smile.

Unless I absolutely had to, I never looked in the direction of the bed on my right. There was something about Ellen which disturbed me. She must have been about my age, a beautiful woman with thick black hair and big dark eyes. She could not speak at all, but communicated with the world by a series of expressive hissing sounds. She was almost completely unable to move and when she was not hissing she sat in her wheelchair gazing into space. On the locker beside her was a photo of her three teenage children and a smiling husband but they never came in to see her. A junior nurse told me she had been like that for almost a year.

'She had the same thing as you,' she said. I shuddered and told myself firmly the nurse must have been mistaken. Ellen was a cripple.

'It's not surprising the health service is short of money,' said a rather tactless visitor of mine as he sat watching the nurses helping her to drink her tea. 'She's just a cabbage really.' Although I did not want to be identified with Ellen in any way, his remark still made me furious.

'Just because you can't speak doesn't mean you can't think and feel,' I retorted, and then realised I would probably have agreed with him a few months before. Now I understood how she felt only too well, and perhaps that was why I had to push her out of my mind. I still would not allow myself to face the fact that my own body was still like a floppy rag doll. Lying flat for so long would make anyone weak, I told

41

myself. However, as the weeks went by, even I could see I was not making progress.

Pain was now a constant part of my life and it was often so bad I spent much of the time being physically sick. It was not just my head, every single part of my body seemed to hurt. When people approached my bed I dreaded their touching me. I would have screamed if they had, providing I could have summoned enough breath. Noise and light became so painful again Sister had my bed shunted into a side ward where I could have the curtains drawn. The peace and quiet helped me greatly, but if it had not been for the chaplain's visits I would never have coped with the loneliness – or the boredom.

On my locker stood a photo of my family and I thought about them continuously as I lay looking at it. Tony brought some of the children in to see me for very short visits, one at a time, but I think we all found that very upsetting. The pain was so severe I was terrified they would jump on the bed or give me one of their bear hugs. The sight of me looking so ill was disturbing and it was hard for them to understand why they could not touch me. Tony's evening visits were the only things which made life worth the effort, but he could never stay for long because it was important to maintain the security of the children's bedtime routine.

One day the neurologist came down from London to see me again.

'Why am I taking so long to get better?' I demanded. 'When I had encephalitis twenty years ago, it wasn't like this at all.' He explained that I had developed a complication. The casings of my nerves had also become inflamed.

'How long will it be before the inflammation dies down?' I asked.

'We just don't know that,' he replied. He wasn't smiling any more as he went on to explain the possibility that the nerves may be left permanently damaged by scarring.

'You mean I might not get completely better?' I felt stunned. He said nothing, but to my great surprise bent down

42

and pulled my bedsocks back on for me. I did not think important consultants ever did things like that.

'Rest,' he said gently. 'That's the best thing you can do at this stage.'

'Of course I'll get better,' I told myself firmly when he had gone. 'He only said there was a "possibility".' Before he came to see me that evening, Tony had rather a depressing interview with Sister. He looked positively crushed when he slumped down in the armchair beside me.

'I'm so much better,' I told him brightly, 'I'll soon be home now to look after you.' I could hear myself sounding like Mrs Pennington encouraging her poor old husband, but I really wanted to say, 'If I'm stuck in a wheelchair like Ellen, will you still go on loving me?' He wanted to talk about the things Sister had said in her office, but somehow neither of us managed to say anything at all. A barrier had come down between us which had never been there before.

The following morning Sister arranged for us to see the hospital social worker and Tony took an hour off work for the interview. He arrived after a long walk through heavy rain, his jacket sodden and his hair plastered to his head. I yearned to make him a hot cup of coffee and give his shirt a quick iron. When the social worker arrived she was an efficient young woman, immaculately dressed, but she gave us the impression that her opinion of men was rather low. Tony did his best all the same.

'I feel I may need some help when Jen comes home,' he began diffidently.

'Oh?' she replied as she arranged the papers in her brief case. 'But you're managing all right now aren't you?'

'Well, I've had to go back to work, of course, but the four-year-old spends the day with the lady who runs the playgroup. She brings him home at teatime and stays for a while so there's someone there when the others come back from school.'

'Oh well, you're all right then,' she said, casually dismissing all the washing, cooking and cleaning – not to mention the outside jobs which go with a self-sufficient life in the country. Tony swallowed hard.

'I don't think I'll be able to nurse Jen on top of everything else,' he said.

'I'm afraid we can't be of any help to you out there in the country. Things are easier in towns. We simply don't have the resources or the funds. You're just going to have to get on with it, I'm afraid. Plenty of other people do.'

'But I've got six children,' said Tony bleakly.

'Don't worry, darling,' I said, when the sound of her high heels had disappeared in the distance. 'I'm going to get better, you'll see. Once I'm home again, I'll be fine.' He did not look convinced as he blundered out of the room on his way back to work.

The day stretched out ahead of me, and the dark, stuffy little room felt like a prison. During the dullest patch of the day (after lunch and before visiting time), the doors swung open with a flourish and in bounded two people in short white tunics. They said they were physiotherapists, but they seemed more like angels of hope to me.

'We'll soon sort you out,' they said cheerfully. 'We've had patients far worse than you are, running round the car park. But you won't like the things we make you do.' They were right there! Shaking my head like a dog after a swim and rolling my eyeballs round in circles were the very last things I wanted to do.

'The pain makes me so giddy,' I explained as I clutched the sick bowl.

'But we *want* to make you giddy,' they explained kindly. 'The brain has to be trained to find new nerve pathways when the old ones are damaged.' When they stood me up by my bed it felt so odd not being able to feel my feet and I frequently crashed to the floor like a felled tree.

Every day after that one of them came in to 'torture' me, and I loved them for it! At last I could do something towards my own recovery, and their sense of humour made everything seem amusing. It was very funny when they told me to place

44

the tip of my finger on the end of my nose and I only succeeded in ramming it right in my eye! After a few days I learnt to balance sufficiently to walk a few steps – so long as I leant well forward and stuck out my backside. I knew I looked like a waddling duck but they laughed *with* me and not *at* me so it did not matter. Their ten-minute visits left me totally exhausted but I did not mind resting when I felt I had earned it.

One afternoon a porter came into my room with a wheelchair.

'You're going down to the physio department today,' he said cheerfully. This was real promotion. To be out in the great world beyond the ward's swing-doors would be a marvellous treat. As we set off, the vertigo was just as unpleasant as ever, but it was no longer terrifying because I'd had plenty of time to get used to it. This time I also took the precaution of asking a nurse to stick Tony's sunglasses firmly to my head with sticky tape.

The lift was full of people from the outside world. I gazed at them and thought how well they all looked. They were the nice ordinary kind who might easily have lived in our village. I had a sudden yearning to talk about absorbing things, such as the effect of the drought on vegetable marrows and the wicked price of French apples. I smiled up at them encouragingly as the lift descended, but for some reason they did not seem to see me, they were all talking to the porter behind me.

Was I invisible, just because I was in a wheelchair? It was a long time since I had looked at myself in a mirror but I was conscious that my face twitched and winked in an unpredictable manner, and the patch which the physios had put over one eye to stimulate the muscles of the other must have made me look a bit odd. I even began to regret the sticky-taped glasses. Concentrating hard on my hands to stop them from shaking I smiled once again. Surely these people must realise that inside I was still a perfectly normal housewife?

'It's a bit hot today,' I said to the woman carrying a bunch of roses. Well that is what I meant to say, actually it sounded more like; 'Icha bitcha ot tomorrow.' She looked embarrassed and hastily turned round to talk to her husband. I was mortified. I wanted to shout, 'There's nothing wrong with my speech usually, I just get a bit muddled when I'm nervous.'

'Does she like grapes?' asked another woman, addressing the porter as if I did not exist. 'My sister's too ill to eat these.'

I was not going to risk speech again so I nodded vigorously and held out my wobbling hands, but she gave them to the porter who hung the bag out of reach on the handle of the chair.

'There you go,' he said as the doors slid open, and before I could make those people realise I was not an imbecile he whisked me away out of sight.

Chapter 5

'If only you'd let me go home, I know I'd be better in a week!'
I was looking up into those nice grey eyes of my favourite
doctor again but for once they were not smiling.

'Sorry, but it's still too soon, Mrs Larcombe.' He was sitting on the side of my bed and as usual he was taking the
time to explain. After two months in the Kent and Sussex
there was nothing more they could do for me and they needed
my bed. Yet I was still not well enough to go home.

'You need at least a month of convalescence in a place
where you can carry on with the physio and have some kind
of counselling and rehabilitation.' I shuddered as I pictured
myself incarcerated in some institution miles from home and
being drilled from dawn by ex-army sergeants, or, worse still
– making basket-work mats.

'It sounds ghastly!' I said.

'Yes, doesn't it,' he replied apologetically.

'There's always Burrswood,' I suggested tentatively, 'but
we'd never afford the fees.'

'Now, why ever didn't I think of Burrswood myself? With
your religious convictions it would be the perfect place, and
it's close to your family as well. We often refer patients there,
so there might well be ways of coping with finance. I'll go
and see what I can fix right now.'

He hurried away, with his crumpled white coat flapping
behind him. Lying back on the pillows I closed my eyes. I
was back in the main ward by then and the hospital noise
seemed to clatter on continuously. I had reached the point

47

when I yearned for peace and privacy like a wilting house plant needs water. In my mind I pictured Burrswood – a large country house attached to a church and surrounded by magnificent gardens. An old school friend of mine worked there, and once she had shown me round. The Christian healing centre, she explained, was a nursing and convalescent home, run by a community of Christians who believed in prayer as well as medicine. She also told me about the remarkable lady who had founded it soon after the Second World War. Dorothy Kerin. When she was a young girl, dying of an incurable disease, she had suddenly and supernaturally recovered. Soon afterwards God spoke to her in a dream and said that he had brought her back 'to heal the sick, comfort the sorrowing and give faith to the faithless'. This had so convinced her of the power of divine healing that she began to pray for the sick herself. She believed that people not only needed prayer and sound medical help when they were ill, but they mended best in beautiful surroundings with plenty of 'tender loving care'. Burrswood was the beautiful result of that insight. I simply could not think of anywhere I would rather go – except home.

At long last the day came when I was due to leave the Kent and Sussex Hospital. I was so excited I was ready hours before Tony came to transport me the five miles to Burrswood. It felt good to be wearing clothes again although the effort of putting them on had been enormous. Tony must have guessed dressing might be a problem because he had arrived the night before with a roll-neck sweater and a skirt with an elastic waistband. The sweater was easy but the skirt presented more of a problem. It was very difficult to pull it on without standing up, but even harder to stand up without any sense of balance! It was putting on the tights, however, which finally reduced me to tears of frustration.

With the help of a nurse I was dressed at long last and feeling quite pleased with my appearance as I sat waiting for Tony. Looking back now I realise I must actually have looked anything but attractive. I had lost so much weight the skirt hung on me like an empty potato sack while the tights sagged and wrinkled round my spindly legs. The eye patch, sticky-taped glasses and National Health walking stick did not make fashionable accessories. Tony came through the swing-doors of the ward and I will never forget the shock on his face. Until then I had always been in bed when he came to visit me. Clothes made the change in me much more obtrusive. I struggled to my feet to meet him, but he stopped short at the end of my bed.

'I can't take you out looking like that,' he hissed.

'Looking like what?' I demanded, and wished my face would stop its endless twitching. I had a nasty feeling I could see revulsion in his eyes.

'At least take that ridiculous sticky tape off your forehead.' We were both angry now. We glared at each other over the hospital bed and the tension did not lessen as we moved off down the corridor. It was the first time Tony had pushed me in a wheelchair and I think the experience was equally difficult for both of us. Walking along with someone whose back is always to you does not make conversation very easy.

Now that the long awaited moment of leaving had arrived I was not so sure I really wanted to go. After so long in hospital I had become institutionalised: a machine, dependent on ward routine, which ate, slept and washed itself at the prescribed times each day – and opened its mouth mechanically at the sight of a pill. The thought of having to learn a whole new set of rules when I arrived at Burrswood was almost unbearable. All I wanted to do was go home with Tony and never see another person in uniform as long as I lived.

The journey should have taken only a few minutes but it was more than an hour before we arrived. The movement of the car was so traumatic that Tony stopped to give me a chance to recover, but he had the sense to drive us into the middle of a wood in order to do so. He knew how much I would love to be surrounded by the cool green shade of the trees and as I sat with my head on his shoulder the gentle

49

sounds of the country soothed us both. But we couldn't stay there for ever, and as we drove up to Burrswood I was shaking violently. Illness has a way of sapping your self-confidence.

The nurse who met us in the hall soon dispersed my anxiety. She even knelt down on the floor so she was at my level (a rare treat for a wheelchair occupant) and shook hands with me. 'We've already been praying that you'll be happy here,' she said. Suddenly I felt like a real person with a mind and emotions, not just a body in need of repair.

The bedroom was so beautiful I could hardly believe it was really intended for me. Antique furniture, pictures, soft carpet, and flowers everywhere. A marked contrast from the polished floors and stark white walls of hospital. I could even hear birds singing outside in the beech trees and see blue hills in the distance.

When they brought in afternoon tea the desire to pour out my own cup was so strong I seized the pot with both hands, but it slithered away from me and deposited its contents all over the tray. I waited cringing for the nurse's wrath, but she merely smiled and fetched some more.

It felt so normal sitting there drinking tea together and looking out over the gardens. 'Surely,' I thought, 'we'll be able to relax and talk to each other properly at last.' Our conversations had been so stilted and rushed in the ward. Even during our interlude in the wood that afternoon Tony still treated me like a fragile china doll that might break at any moment. That barrier was still between us and he kept looking restlessly at his watch.

'I really ought to get home and see how Sarah is coping with supper,' he said, and soon he disappeared. At long last I allowed the smile I had worn for months to slide from my face and I cried for well over an hour.

The following morning, after the heady delights of being lowered into the bath by a 'crane' and then having my hair cut and set, I was pushed into the chapel for the healing service. These are held several times a week and people come from all over the country to attend. My expectations were high because I was convinced that prayer would speed my recovery and send me home completely fit. Perhaps I would even be healed instantly like Dorothy Kerin. Sometimes it happens at Burrswood. I have to admit that my nonconformist background made me feel a little out of place in the chapel; we did not have statues, candles and robed clergymen in our church. The tune of the first hymn, however, was one of my favourites and I began to relax. So it was rather a blow when I discovered that my chest muscles were too weak to allow me to sing. Those of us in wheelchairs were parked in the aisle and Father Keith, the chaplain, came to pray for us first before the rest of the congregation walked up to the communion rail. For some reason I thought I would feel intensely embarrassed as he put his hands on my head, but when he smiled down at me he had one of the kindest faces I had ever seen. His prayer was beautiful too.

'Please let it work,' I echoed inwardly.

It would have been lovely to spend all my time out in the beautiful gardens, enjoying the roses and the views of those distant hills. Unfortunately my eyes could not tolerate the bright summer sunlight, but one afternoon when it was rather grey and overcast a nurse offered to wheel me out for an airing.

At the end of the terrace sat another patient.

'I'll park your chair next to her,' said the nurse brightly. Usually I am gregarious by nature, but I was still feeling embarrassed about my odd speech and the ridiculous way my face and hands kept twitching. I would have preferred to be alone to look at the garden in peace but it was a little too late by then to say so.

'This is our Madge,' said the nurse. In hospital people were often referred to as 'the angina' or 'the Parkinson's', but at Burrswood Madge was herself and not just 'the multiple sclerosis'. Soon she had produced the inevitable photos of her children and I swapped them with mine. It was easier, I soon discovered, to talk to someone else in a wheelchair: our

51

eyes were on the same level and she too sounded rather drunk when she talked!

'I come here every summer for two weeks' holiday,' she told me, and went on to explain that she lived in a Cheshire Home with twenty other disabled people.

'But your family . . .' I faltered, 'all those children.'

'You'll have to learn that ninety per cent of marriages break up when one partner suddenly becomes disabled.'

'Surely that's exaggerated,' I protested.

'You obviously haven't been disabled for very long,' she commented drily.

'Oh but I'm not disabled at all,' I corrected her. 'I've only been ill.'

'Really?' she said in a tone which I found rather irritating.

I looked back at her photos and found one of her husband at the helm of a yacht and another of him climbing the side of a rock face. He looked a nice man. 'How could he possibly put . . . ?'

'Put me into an institution?' she finished. 'He didn't, it was my decision. I got sick and tired of trying to keep up with the able-bodied world. It's a lot less stressful and a lot more companionable being with your own kind. You'll discover that too,' she added. 'And what's more you owe it to your family.' I must have looked puzzled because she continued, 'What's a person to do when they're still young and full of energy but they have to watch their partner gradually becoming prematurely old and decrepit? Should they chuck away their own youth too? Should they stop going off sailing for the weekend or out in the evenings just because their partners need someone with them all the time, to dress them, feed them and empty their smelly catheter? No, if we don't make it easy for them to leave, we force them to become disabled along with us.'

'Her family must be selfish monsters,' I thought.

'Don't look so worried,' she said. 'We have a lot of fun in the home. If you want to be a successful disabled person, you've got to be willing to let go of the old life and all the things you can't do – and start enjoying the things you can do.'

After that I carefully avoided Madge. I was going to get better, and my mind was closed to any alternative way of living.

Almost every day I had a visit from one of the Burrswood doctors. He was a gentle old Scotsman who did me far more good by describing his beloved lochs and salmon rivers than ever he did by his medicine. On only one occasion did he attempt to help me look at the future honestly.

'You do realise, don't you,' he said when he came to my room one hot afternoon in late July, 'that you will need full-time help when you get home.' I looked at him in disbelief as he continued, 'You'll be needing someone to look after you as well as the children.'

'But the social services can't offer us any help at all,' I told him, 'and we couldn't even afford a cleaner for an hour a week.' I had to smile when I thought how much we would have to pay the kind of nurse-cook-gardener-chauffeur-nanny-char he was describing. Even if we had been million-aires I would not have been willing to hand over my household to someone else; our privacy was too important.

'I've just got to get better quickly,' I told him airily. 'After all, I've got a whole month here, that's sure to be enough time.'

'It will be at least eighteen months until we can tell how things are going to turn out in the long term,' he said omin-ously. 'Rest will make recovery more likely.'

'He's a dear,' I told myself as he returned to his fishing stories, 'but he is a bit old fashioned. Nowadays we fight for recovery, pushing ourselves to the limit each day. We don't sit about resting. Housework and gardening will be good physiotherapy for me.'

At first I positively basked in all the luxury and care offered at Burrswood and I felt deeply grateful to the people in our church who had clubbed together to pay all the fees, but as I grew stronger I began to miss the children too much to enjoy anything without them. When they came to see me they still seemed very strained and distant. At the time I found that hard to understand. Now I realise it was because they found the change in me such a shock.

It was also about that time that everything at home seemed to be going badly wrong. The lady who had been looking after Richard each day was no longer able to help after her father had a stroke. Richard had to spend each day with a different set of people, which was very bewildering for a small child. The strain of making sure the others were all collected from different schools and catered for to the end of the day was also taking its toll on Tony. It was not even as if he could relax with them when he arrived home from work because he felt it was important to keep up their personal interests and activities. Justyn, who was then thirteen and passionately fond of sport, was in training for the National Swimming Championships. That meant two training sessions a day. Tony would get up at five, do the twenty-mile round trip with him to the pool in Tunbridge Wells, dash home, help Sarah get the younger ones up, dressed, fed and off to school. Then he would drive back to work, shop in his lunch hour and hurry home to supervise tea.

The chores were endless and someone always needed to be taken to Brownies or a music lesson. Then the boys had to be settled in bed before he was free to take Justyn back for his evening training session. If he was lucky, he fitted in a trip to see me somewhere in the middle of all that. It was a gruelling regime and would have been an impossible one without Sarah. She had grown up overnight, as she stepped into my shoes and became the 'hub' of the family. But for a fourteen-year-old, the sheer mountain of responsibility and hard work was really far too much on top of school. Sometimes she was still up doing her homework at midnight.

At first friends and neighbours offered Tony a lot of help, but it is difficult for people to commit themselves on a long-term basis, and after a while they naturally began to drift back to their own lives again. They said, 'Do let us know if you need anything.' But somehow it was easier for Tony to do the jobs himself than spend hours on the phone fixing things up and then having to be grateful afterwards.

Well-meaning friends came over to Burrswood in the afternoons to drink tea with me and tell me 'how worried' they were about him.

'On the point of a breakdown,' they said.

He is fiercely independent and, like the horse in George Orwell's *Animal Farm*, his motto in difficult situations is always, 'I will work harder.' But the horse died of exhaustion in the end.

When he managed to come in to see me his face was grey and expressionless with fatigue. (He looked like someone who has had a massive haemorrhage.) All his vitality and strength seemed to have drained away.

'How are things really?' I would ask anxiously, to which he would always reply, 'Everything's fine', but I knew that was not true. He was merely shielding me from worry. Some people talk about their problems at length and seem to mend themselves by doing so. Tony is one of those who crawls away with his into an emotional 'hole' and hides there with them silently. I could see he was living in a personal nightmare and I would have given anything I possessed to help or comfort him. So his silence infuriated me until I nagged and needled him every time he came near me. I could hear myself doing it, I knew it would make things even worse for him, but still I seemed incapable of stopping myself.

My visitors were much more forthcoming with their information. They told me Jane, who was then twelve, was becoming unable to communicate with anyone and so withdrawn she spent most of her time locked in her bedroom. That did not surprise me: every adult she had ever loved and trusted seemed destined to let her down.

Visitors also told me Duncan was totally out of hand. That was more difficult to understand. We had nicknamed him 'The Badger' because at six he was such a quiet, good-natured person. When people said he was rude and angry with anyone who offered him friendship, they seemed to be talking about a different child from the one I knew. When friends asked him to tea after school he refused to eat anything and promptly ran away. While they frantically searched the village he would be sitting on our front doorstep waiting for Tony to come home. He had always loved school, but now they told me he could not sit still and his restless disruptive behaviour was driving his poor teacher mad. I hated to think of him making himself so objectionable at a time when he most needed love and acceptance.

The one joy of his life was the yellow budgie I had given him for his last birthday. He used to let it fly round his bedroom and even coaxed it to perch on his finger. One day the cat jumped out from under his bed and killed the little bird before he could do anything to save it. He is perhaps the most sensitive of all the children and I was desperate to be able to comfort and reassure him. The frustration of sitting there impotent in the middle of all that luxury was intolerable.

'Do bring him in to see me,' I pleaded with Tony, but he was hesitant. Duncan and Jane were the only two he had not yet brought in to visit me, simply because they did not seem very keen to come. Duncan had been ill for the first two years of his life and so often in hospital that anything in a white coat still terrified him. 'He might feel happier if he saw how lovely Burrswood is,' I pointed out. 'Surely he just needs some reassurance from me.' I continued to nag until Tony finally relented.

Duncan came one day after tea. I watched him climb out of the car from my bedroom window and as he walked to the front door his legs were so stiff with excitement he seemed to have no knees at all. He looked as gorgeous as only a blue-eyed six-year-old can, but someone had brushed his hair into a new style and he was wearing a shirt I had not bought for him. He had grown thinner and taller and for some reason he did not seem *mine* any more. As the door opened I wanted to run across and hug him, tell him I'd soon be home to make everything just as lovely as it always had been. But, as I struggled to stand up, he stopped and stared at me balefully and then backed himself into a corner.

'If I talk to him soothingly,' I thought, 'he'll soon settle down.' But because I was agitated the words came out in a tangled, unintelligible mess. When I lurched across the room towards him he began to hurl everything from the top of the chest of drawers on to the floor. Tony hastily tried to restrain him, and he began to kick and bellow furiously. A nurse hurried in looking horrified.

'It's all right,' said Tony grimly, 'we're just leaving.' And they did. As I watched the car disappear round the corner I felt quite devastated. In fact I was so upset they called the doctor, who said my pulse was racing at a dangerously high speed. He put me on drugs to regulate it but they made me feel so exhausted the physiotherapy had to be stopped.

'I'm going backwards not forwards,' I thought in despair. 'I'll never get home to them all at this rate.'

The old sense of guilt that I had always had about illness began to press me down like a heavy load of lead in a rucksack. It must have been something I had done which had brought all this misery on my family but whatever was it? My visitors provided plenty of answers – my vegetarian diet, our rustic drainage system or the large size of our family.

'We did warn you,' said one of them as she handed me some sweet peas from her garden. 'Doing too much; that's what brought all this on, fostering children and dashing round the village like a mad thing – we could all see it coming but you wouldn't listen.' I couldn't blame them, because I too had always looked for causes. When a neighbour about my age had a heart attack, I had thought, 'I'm not surprised, she was so overweight.' A local vicar had a stroke and I joined everyone else by saying he worried too much. Perhaps we are all basically afraid of illness so we feel more comfortable if we can convince ourselves that 'it could never happen to me' because we are so careful about the way we live. But it *had* happened to me, and feeling guilty about it was not helping my recovery.

'Just rest dear,' the nurses told me. 'Try not to worry about your children. Do some jigsaw puzzles – they'll help your hand and eye co-ordination.'

'I don't want to sit here doing puzzles, when my kids need me at home,' I thought one hot afternoon, as those silly little pieces refused to be picked up by my floppy fingers. So I chucked the whole lot over the floor. Doing that did not make me feel any better!

That evening Father Keith knocked at the door of my room. 'They tell me you're not doing so well,' he said, as he pulled a stool up to my chair. 'Is something worrying you?' Out it all gushed, the self-condemnation and the anxiety about the family.

He listened to it all without a single interruption and then very quietly he said, 'You're carrying such a lot of guilt about with you, aren't you? I don't think you have anything to feel guilty about at all, but the fact that you do is what counts. Why don't you just put it down at the foot of Christ's cross? That's the reason he allowed himself to be nailed there wasn't it.' Somehow as Father Keith knelt silently beside me, it felt just as if that heavy rucksack was slipping off my back at long last.

'But what can I do for Tony and the children?' I asked him after a while. 'I sit here praying for them but nothing seems to penetrate the ceiling.'

'Perhaps you need to pray in a more tangible kind of a way,' he said thoughtfully. 'It sounds as if they all need a touch of God's healing. Trauma can wound the spirit and the mind like a car accident wounds the body.'

'But we'd never get them here to a healing service.' I had a mental picture of a team of sheep dogs trying to round them up and I wondered what Duncan would do to the candles in that ornate chapel.

'They don't have to come here for prayer,' said Father Keith, and he produced from his pocket a little bottle of oil. 'Give me your hands,' he said, and poured a few drops into each palm. Then to my embarrassment he knelt down again by my chair. 'You lay your hands on my head,' he said, 'and I will represent Tony and all the children while you pray.'

'But I can't do that,' I protested. I was positively cringing. 'I don't have a gift of healing and you're a priest.'

He looked up and smiled at me. 'When I touch the sick people down in the chapel, it isn't my hands that heal them, but the power of God flowing through my hands. He can just as easily use your hands as mine. I'm no more "worthy" than you – none of us is ever worthy to be used by God but he uses us just the same.' Then he bent his head again and seemed to be waiting for me to begin. I felt so silly praying out loud in front of a man like him, but after a few moments I forgot he was even there as I poured everything out to God in a jumble of words only he could possibly understand. At the end I was so exhausted I lay back in the chair and for a long while Father Keith continued to kneel beside me motionless. The peace I experienced that evening is something I will never forget.

When Tony next came to see me he looked different. I don't think the situation actually became any easier but he seemed to be coping better and the children were definitely happier and more settled. When the school holidays arrived they all went off to Yorkshire and had a holiday in a Quaker hostel. I hated their going without me, but I knew I would be going home as soon as they arrived back. Just that thought alone was enough to keep me going.

Chapter 6

Sitting in that beautiful bedroom at Burrswood, I must have planned every detail of my return home a thousand times over. I pictured myself bustling into the house, unpacking in my own familiar bedroom and then having a good spring-clean – the house was sure to resemble a rubbish tip. Then I'd cook a delicious meal and we'd all sit round the table, catching up on news before I put the little ones to bed. In my daydreams I genuinely saw myself stepping back into my life again at the point where it had been interrupted. I was much stronger by then and mobile enough to manage without the wheelchair. I still walked like an inebriated duck, waddling from one piece of furniture to another, but I did not realise that at the time. I even thought I would be able to manage without sticks when I went home. As I looked round the chapel I felt positively sprightly in comparison with the other Burrswood inmates.

'Are you feeling confident about going home?' asked Father Keith when he came to say goodbye at the end of my stay.

'Oh yes,' I replied, 'after all those services and so much prayer I'm sure I'll be fine once I settle back into the routine.' He put a hand on my bony shoulder and said quietly,

'Prayer isn't dictating to God what we want. It's taking time to know what God wants and then gaining the strength to do it.'

'Oh but I'm sure God would want me to be perfectly well,' I said. 'Once in the hospital, I nearly died and I'm sure I was "told" I would recover.' Father Keith looked down at me silently, and then he smiled.

'Always hold on to that,' he said, 'whatever happens.' So, on a cloud of hope and good intentions, I went home.

It was a hot August afternoon when we began to be a family again and it could not have been more different from the way I imagined. It was the middle of the school holidays so Tony was at home – but so were all the children. I had forgotten just how much noise they made. After the journey I discovered I was far too tired to think about unpacking, and my friend Grace had already spring-cleaned the house.

'What shall I cook you for dinner?' I asked Tony brightly as I tottered towards the kitchen, but because I could not feel where my feet were I tripped straight over the rug in the hall. I needed those walking sticks more than I realised! Undeterred I began to clatter about the kitchen making 'busy' noises to indicate that I was back in my old position once again. But I was somewhat deflated when I discovered I could not find anything. Sarah had reorganised all my drawers and cupboards.

'Why?' I demanded furiously.

'It took her a whole day to do it,' said Tony reproachfully. 'She thought it would be a lovely surprise. You could at least be grateful.' I felt ridiculously threatened, as if they were both ganging up on me and criticising the way I had previously arranged everything.

Lying in bed at Burrswood it had seemed so easy to produce a meal, but when faced with the reality I discovered something seemed to have gone wrong with my ability to think, and I could not remember the way to cook even the simplest of things. I reached for the frying pan and found my hands were too weak to lift it. When I tried to chop an onion it slithered away from me, and left me to slice my fingers instead. They did not hurt, because I had little feeling in my limbs and I could not think where all the blood was coming from. This lack of sensation made hot dishes hazardous and I was surprised when I watched the blisters appear.

Long before the meal was ready that day, I sat down in despair and left Tony and Sarah to clear the chaos I had created.

'I'm just tired after the journey,' I told them firmly.

When they finally dished up the dinner it was not the leisurely affair I had pictured either. It was so long since I had sat at a table and eaten a meal with other people, I found the experience shattering. Sound was still a problem for me and when everyone talked at once their voices were distorted into a painful roar. My muscles were too weak to produce enough voice to compete successfully. When I did begin to speak I muddled things like 'his' and 'hers' and 'up' and 'down' or forgot a vital word in mid sentence. I wanted to communicate with them so badly, but at first they looked at me blankly. That could have caused me great anguish but when I managed to tell Richard to hurry up and 'sit on' his fish fingers Justyn suddenly began to laugh. Even though he was so strong and well co-ordinated physically, right from the start he treated me with a tenderness and understanding which was extraordinary for a boy of thirteen. He laughed at me often but in the kind of way which made me feel that, to him, my limitations were unimportant and even endearing. During that first meal I realised that allowing my oddities to become a family joke would prevent the children from realising how much they worried me.

As the day progressed it became increasingly hard to keep cheerful. Sarah's heavy metal pop competed with Naomi's Beethoven symphonies and the boys argued loudly over television programmes. I began to wonder how I was going to cope. They all seemed to move so fast, darting about the house like swallows catching gnats. It all made me so giddy I huddled on the sofa, terrified they would bump into me. The light, too, was a terrible problem; I longed to close the curtains and block out the bright sunshine.

At long last it was bedtime and I crawled thankfully upstairs on my hands and knees.

'What on earth are you doing?' demanded Tony incredulously as I rooted in my drawers for woolly tights, winter vests and thick jumpers.

'I'm frozen,' I told him through my chattering teeth. 'Please, couldn't we have the windows closed?'

'But we're right in the middle of a heat wave,' he protested. 'I'll cook if we don't have some air.' As time went on, the damage to my heat regulating mechanism often caused great hilarity. Being hot when everyone else was cold, and cold when they were hot, made me feel out of phase with the rest of humanity.

When we finally climbed into bed Tony was so tired he was asleep within seconds. That first day must have been as hard for him as it was for me, but he never said anything about the way he felt. By that time he was past the stage of treating me like a fragile doll. He never fussed, wrapped me in cotton wool or tried to help me unless I asked. Onlookers might even have thought he was unfeeling, but actually his detached approach helped as much as Justyn's laughter to restore my self-confidence.

As I lay thankfully in the dark and stillness of the night I did some serious thinking. To exist comfortably at home I would have to sentence the children to a life of sitting motionless in semi-darkness without making a sound. Of course that was out of the question – they would have all wished I was back in hospital. I was just going to have to pretend I was fine and not let anyone know about the discomforts of my private world. Talking about symptoms of any kind was something I was going to have to try to avoid.

Early next morning I woke half expecting a night nurse to check my pulse. When I realised I was actually at home, it was a wave of panic and not relief which pushed me back under the bedclothes. Tony was already down in the kitchen and when he appeared with a cup of tea, I felt oddly embarrassed, as if we were strangers. We sipped our tea in a rather strained silence, and as usual I reached for my diary. In handwriting which looked as if it had been formed by a demented spider I scrawled an urgent prayer: 'August 1982   Oh God

63

please help me to be good tempered today.' Later, probably the following morning, I added a rather disillusioned foot-note, 'I wasn't!'

Actually I was unbearably cross, and the more I tried to stop myself the worse I became. The three girls were due to go away to various camps and it never occurred to me not to help them pack their kit. Surely mothers always do? Perhaps the pain was extra bad that day, or maybe I just wanted to show them I was still the boss. Anyway, after an hour of getting in their way I was being so unpleasant Sarah was looking thunderous, Jane was in tears and Naomi said sweetly, 'Mummy, why don't you just sit down for a while and I'll make you a nice cup of coffee?'

'But you're all in a total mess,' I exploded. 'This family has gone wild like the garden since I left; now I'm back I've got to sort you out somehow!'

'We managed fine while you were away,' said Sarah furiously. 'Dad relied on me for everything and we all knew exactly what we were supposed to do. Now you're home you're just upsetting everything.'

As I was drinking my coffee, Duncan came running in from the garden, his nose streaming with blood. Once he would have come to me for comfort, but he ran straight to Sarah. Suddenly I felt redundant and almost like an intruder. At Burrswood I had thought it would make life easier for them when I got home, but I was creating more work because I still needed so much help.

'Never mind,' I thought confidently, 'the more I do the sooner I'll be better.' This resolve, however, presented Tony with quite a dilemma. For instance, I wanted to feel 'in control' by helping produce the meals and dishing out the food at table. What I did not realise was that I now operated at the pace of an elderly tortoise. While he was madly dashing about trying to cater for so many children who moved at high speed, the last thing he needed was me dropping eggs on the floor and spilling milk over the table. Yet he did not feel he could crush me by saying I was in his way.

So he allowed me to go on with the illusion that I was getting better all the time and would soon be perfectly fit. It was not until the day Richard started school that my 'make believe' world finished abruptly.

Handing a five-year-old over to the reception class teacher is a symbolic moment in a mother's life so I insisted on taking Richard to school that September morning. It was also the first time I had been up to the village and I was longing to see all my friends again at the school gate. That was the place where all the gossip was exchanged. But as I walked slowly across the car park holding Tony's arm and Richard's hand I was conscious of eyes staring at me from all directions. Normally I would have bounced into the centre of the group of mums demanding to know everyone's news but suddenly I felt shy and painfully conscious of a body which was not quite under my control. It must have been a bit of a shock for them, I suppose, because I weighed at least four stones less than when they had last seen me. Some people smiled, but I saw pity in their eyes, while others turned hurriedly away and pretended they had not seen us at all. I am not sure which reaction hurt the more.

Friends have often told me how hard they found it to appear in public for the first time after a bereavement or some other kind of major trauma. No one quite knows what to say to them, so they cross the road or hurry into a shop to avoid having to make contact. Perhaps that is only because nowadays we fear illness and death so much we prefer to ignore them and we instinctively shy away from other people's suffering.

This embarrassed reaction made me feel terribly excluded and as I looked at the crowd round the gate of the school playground I suddenly thought, 'I don't fit in with them now. I'm not a real mum any more.'

That night at supper Duncan capped it all when he said to me, 'Don't ever come up to school again, will you? I don't like my friends staring at you.' Probably the hardest part of being disabled is the moment when you first realise that you are.

Not everyone ignored me, of course. Many people were only too anxious to be helpful, but I am ashamed to say I found that almost as disturbing.

'We'll organise a rota for the housework and ironing,' they suggested. The thought appalled me. The last thing I wanted was half the neighbourhood organising my household, washing our underclothes and thinking of us as the official village 'problem'. So I firmly refused their offers of help – I had become the kind of prickly disabled person I had always found so irritating in the past. I suppose I was walking a tightrope really. I needed help but my self-worth could only be maintained by being allowed to do as much as I could manage. Tony understood that completely, and although help would have made life much easier for him, he was actually wise enough to let me discover my limitations the hard way. It took only a few weeks before I was delighted to allow two kind aunts to pay for a daily help.

It seems hardly surprising that my diary soon announced, 'I'm going off my head with loneliness.' I deserved to be: I snubbed everyone who came near me. I also missed Richard intensely but was not now able to fill the vacuum with a flurry of village affairs. Reading was impossible because my eyes would not focus and I could not even concentrate long enough to follow the soaps on TV. All I seemed to do was flutter about the house all day, arguing ineptly with the vacuum cleaner or smashing the ornaments as I flapped at them with a duster. I could not even do the mending; my fingers refused to hold a darning needle. After years of frenetic activity, boredom was a new sensation.

'September 10th   What am I supposed to do all day? By ten in the morning I think the clock must have stopped.' I remember standing on our patio looking over the fields one morning and wondering if the blackberries were ripe in the hedgerows yet. The village still nestled itself round the church on the hill and it would be humming with all the usual autumn events, but I felt left behind – like someone forced unwillingly to retire at only thirty-nine.

Of course I know it was my own fault. The decision to be 'just fine thanks', to anyone who asked must have been infuriating for my friends. Plenty of people trekked all the way down the lane to visit me, but often, when I heard the doorbell, I hid! I did not want people to see what a mess we were in, and it was too difficult to concentrate on a conversation.

Another entry in my diary reads: 'Feel as if my mind has been broken – don't want people to know.' How naïve I was to think I could deceive them! After they had knocked at my door in vain a few times most people took the hint and stopped coming. Just a very few refused to be put off, and they became the friends I relied on down through the years.

At night in my dreams I always seemed to be searching for something or someone I had lost. Was I mourning for my lost body, energy and abilities? Once I dreamed we were at Petworth Place, a National Trust property we loved to visit. Somehow I got myself locked in a cupboard under the stairs. It was so small I could not move my arms or legs and outside I could hear Duncan trying to find me. I can remember still the terrible moment when I heard him begin to scream as he had done that day at Burrswood. I did not even have enough breath to shout to him. In those dreams I felt as devastated as if I had been bereaved.

The doctor at Burrswood had been perfectly right about resting. All my attempted activity simply increased the inflammation, and soon the pain had returned to a viciously high level. Had I known at the time that pain would become a continuous part of everyday life I expect I would have thrust my head into my electric oven and wished it was gas.

'What you two need is a nice romantic weekend in a good hotel a long way from the children,' said Penny our Minister's wife, and she even made it possible by having all our children to stay.

The little holiday began well enough. We drove off towards Dorset early on Saturday morning feeling lightheaded with freedom. It was fourteen years since we had been away alone together and Tony had bought me a new moss-green skirt to celebrate.

'You ought to have something to wear which actually fits you,' he had said when he presented it to me. I felt elegant enough to face any hotel, however grand.

It was one of those misty autumn mornings that hurt you inside with their sheer golden perfection and when we were passing some beech woods I begged Tony to stop. He managed to drive right up a track and suddenly I was surrounded by trees for the first time since the day we drove to Burrswood. I will never forget the way the morning sunlight played on the cobwebs, transforming the drops of dew into strings of ethereal diamonds. We tottered a few yards from the car and then we noticed the toadstools. Little clumps of an unusual variety poked up through the moss all around our feet. Glistening white on long slender stems, they looked as delicate as if they had been Dresden china. We sat down on a fallen tree to enjoy them and savour the rich smell of the earth. This weekend was going to restore us both; that's what Penny had said and I began to agree with her until I realised something awful was happening. My incontinence pad was leaking. I pulled myself up and examined my beautiful new skirt. It was saturated. I had to change behind a bush and face arriving at the hotel in my old sack with the elastic waist. I can laugh now, but at the time my sense of humour deserted me. As we bumped our way off down the track the toadstools and cobwebs ceased to exist for me.

It is often not until you stop that you realise just how tired you actually are. When we were finally shown into our luxurious hotel bedroom Tony flopped on to the bed and slept practically the whole weekend. He had finally succumbed to the months of strain and overwork.

I was so giddy after the journey and in so much pain I swallowed as many pills as I dared and promptly joined him!

It had been Penny's idea that we would have time to talk through our new situation. As she dashed around looking after all those children I wonder what she would have said if she had seen us snoring away our precious time.

Chapter 7

The realisation that I was suffering from depression on top of everything else was the ultimate humiliation. A few days after our weekend away I wrote, 'September 1982   I feel buried deep in the ground under piles of heavy, damp sand. Awful suffocating darkness. Life is pointless, useless and wearily boring. The physical pain and other problems I could put up with, but this *depression* is worse than anything else in the whole world.'

Unwittingly I had always rather despised depressed people, feeling they could, 'jolly well pull themselves together if they tried hard enough'. Discovering I was wrong probably did me a great deal of good. I would have given anything to have been able to pull myself together, and the combination of anxiety and despair is difficult to describe. This is the best description I can give: cowering under the bedclothes, unable to face the day because you don't know if you should wear a dress or a skirt. Then realising life is so pointless it makes no difference what you wear anyway.

'Now I'm going mad on top of everything else,' I thought, and hoped Tony would think I was crying only because the pain was bad. I would not have dreamed of telling him I was depressed. He had quite enough to cope with already.

If only I had not been so pigheaded I would have gone to the doctor, but I did not want to be permanently branded in my medical records as a 'mental patient'. Had I gone he would have been able to reassure me by pointing out that most people who go through bereavement or serious illness become depressed for a while at some stage of their adjustment. Perhaps if I had gone to our Minister he might also have explained that one of the symptoms of depression is this feeling of being abandoned by God.

By that time the Almighty certainly seemed to have disappeared over the far horizon. From the very first day I arrived home from Burrswood I began to feel he could not really love me after all. He had failed to answer all those prayers to make me well again. Ever since childhood I had always known he was the security at the very centre of my existence. Now, just when I needed him most, he was gone. For me, his absence was the worse part of the whole unpleasant situation.

Because I felt I could no longer address God direct, I began writing him messages in a notebook, some of which positively scorched the paper: 'October 1982   Lord, I'm in hell . . . I thought I'd be all right. I thought you'd healed me. I didn't know anything could be as ghastly as this. I'm lost in a wilderness. *Where are you?*'

It was the feeling that I would never now achieve anything worthwhile in life which really got to me. My great aunt's missionary zeal had always goaded me into thinking that I should. Instead I was nothing but a burden on my family and an inconvenience to society.

One day a clergyman friend of ours rang to ask if he could 'pop in' and see me that afternoon. I guessed our friends had put him up to the visit. Obviously people thought I was in need of spiritual guidance, and they were right. So instead of raking furiously for an excuse to put him off, I said a meek, 'Thank you,' and hung up.

It was a bad day for pain, I remember, and for once I had actually succumbed and crawled back to bed. As I lay there waiting for the 'pastoral visit', I wondered if I dared tell him exactly how I really felt. A week before, a friend had taken me back to visit Burrswood. I wanted so badly to tell someone there about the depression, but when it came to the point I was too embarrassed to mention it. Perhaps it was time I finally unzipped myself.

When two o'clock arrived I heard a heavy tread on the stairs and loud clearings of the throat. There was a chair close to the bed, but instead he chose the one farthest away from me, in the extreme corner of the room.

'And how are you?' he asked as if he did not really expect me to tell him. But I did. I spared him nothing – not even the inconvenience.

Once I managed to get myself rolling, it did not seem so hard after all.

'So you see I'm just a physical and mental cripple,' I finished breathlessly. The word 'cripple' appears many times in my diaries before that day, but I had never spoken it out loud before, and hearing it gave me a distinct shock. He laughed as if I were joking.

'Oh I wouldn't say that,' he added bracingly. He ignored all my references to depression as if it was not worth mentioning and said, 'Tell me about this pain then, how bad is it – *really*?' Somehow he conveyed the impression that he did not believe it existed. I tried to describe what it felt like to consider every movement before you made it, to decide whether scratching your nose or drinking a cup of tea were going to be worth the ensuing pain. I did my best, to explain the frustration of knowing that something which filled your entire consciousness was actually quite invisible to other people. They could never understand why living was so difficult for you. While I was talking he ran through what was obviously his range of sympathetic noises.

'Dear, dear, dear,' he said when I ground to a halt, and he still sounded slightly amused. 'But I know just what you mean,' he added. 'I once had a headache which lasted all day.'

It was then that I decided I would never ever talk about pain again. Few people can understand. They either think you are exaggerating for attention, unnerve you with too much sympathy, or they fear pain so much themselves they simply cannot cope and slide hastily away. That clergyman certainly helped me learn that to live successfully with constant pain you have to be a very good actor indeed.

'We all have these low patches,' he said glancing at his watch. 'Try and be more positive. Think about other people a bit more.' It was very good advice, but it came a few months too soon. It was rather like advising an accident victim who is bleeding on the road to 'take a brisk walk round the block'. At a later stage of his recovery exercise would do him a power of good, but at first it would be quite beyond him. Looking back now I can see it was the same with my depression.

'I am sure your faith must be a great help to you,' he said as he rose to leave, and I did not bother to disagree with him.

If only it had been Father Keith in whom I had confided, because once again I was constantly feeling responsible for the bad effect my illness was having on the children. It was only the depression preventing me from thinking rationally, but I am sure he would have helped once again to cope with that guilt. He would also have encouraged me to pray instead of worrying, and I certainly had plenty to worry about.

Duncan's behaviour, far from settling down when I came home, was becoming worse and his whole personality seemed to have changed. Something had broken between us that day at Burrswood and, however hard I tried, I simply did not seem to be able to mend our relationship. He found my disabilities infuriating, and constantly hid my sticks or bit pieces out of my surgical collar. Jane had become uncharacteristically aggressive and Sarah's school work was suffering badly. She later developed school phobia and was unable to go there at all for months at a stretch. Between all six of them they managed to produce enough insecure behaviour to provide material for a whole textbook on disturbed children. We were faced with nightmares, bed-wetting, truancy, shop-lifting, hyper-activity, eating problems, and many other things besides. It was all quite overwhelming, coming as it did when Tony and I were also struggling with our own emotional reactions. We both retreated farther and farther into silence, which probably left the children more bewildered than ever.

They say kids are marvellously resilient, but I think their ability to cope with difficult situations depends a great deal on the way the adults they trust are reacting to those same difficulties. So what chance did ours have with two tense, frozen-faced parents? As we were sitting round the kitchen table having supper one evening in October, Sarah suddenly said,

'We never seem to laugh at mealtimes any more, do we.' The next day I found the sleeping pills.

Opening a drawer, I discovered it was stuffed full of my mother's possessions. She had died not long before, and somehow I could never face disposing of these last few personal oddments. The large bottle of Mogadon was lying there among the diaries and photos. I sat staring at it for a long time. How easy it would be just to go to sleep and never be woken by pain again. It would also be the kindest thing to do for the family – Tony could marry again and provide a nice new mum to look after them all.

Horrified I threw them back in the drawer, but next morning I wrote, 'October 1982   I am lost. Life is quite hopeless. Why didn't I just die that night in June when I had the chance? Tony . . . would be happier without me. I am just a useless zombie. Perhaps I should destroy myself before I damage them any more.' And the day after that, 'I'm hanging over the edge of a precipice, clinging on by my finger nails.'

Those Mogadon seemed to chase me round the house constantly. I thought about them so much I realised at last that I needed professional help – and quickly. It was not so easy to think of a way of getting it confidentially. Whenever I needed to go out, I had to ask someone to take me, and that involved explanations. Then I realised I had an outpatient's appointment at the Kent and Sussex the following week. Perhaps I should tell the consultant how I was feeling, and I could even see the hospital chaplain again at the same time.

He had been such a good friend – sitting quietly by my bed – he was the kind of man who might understand.

For some reason those hospital appointments always had a disastrous effect on both Tony and me: we usually had a massive row in the waiting room, conducted in furious whispers. Perhaps it was the frustration of building up our hopes for weeks that at last the specialist might be able to suggest a cure, and then having to wait most of the day in order to be told there was nothing anyone could do.

That day the consultant was already behind with his appointment list when my name was called, and the sister explained on the way into his room that he had to be in London by three o'clock. He did not look up when I shuffled in and the two medical students who sat beside him did not smile either.

'How are you Mrs . . . er?' he enquired at last, still reading the papers on his desk. I wanted to say 'Terrible. If you don't do something for me soon, I'm not going to go on living,' but instead I heard myself say,

'Fine thanks.'

'That's excellent, excellent. Keep up the good work then. See you in three months.' Doctors invariably have that effect on me!

Tony did not seem to think it was odd when I said I wanted to see the chaplain – alone. He must have suspected something was wrong, however, because I was shaking so violently by the time I knocked on the door marked 'Chaplain'. The Reverend George Swannell was my last hope. If he told me to 'take a more positive attitude', I would go home and swallow every pill I could find.

I remember his little office being terribly dark. Probably it wasn't really, but all my memories of those days seem to be of varying shades of grey. He jumped up from his desk and hurried over towards me. He did not need to say 'how are you?' he just seemed to know.

'I'm terribly sorry,' I began, 'but I seem to have gone into some kind of a depression.' I waited for him to brush that aside like the last clergyman, but instead he sat down beside me and took my hand.

'You must feel absolutely ghastly,' he said gently.

'And I seem to have lost God,' I admitted tentatively, bracing myself for a lecture.

'Well you're in very good company,' was all George said. 'The Lord Jesus felt like that, too, when he was on the cross. He shouted out in the darkness, "My God, my God, why have you forsaken me?" But God is always there even when we don't feel him.'

I do not know whether it was what George said, or the prayer that he prayed for me, but I went home feeling very much better. Maybe it was simply feeling understood. It had been the same that other awful time in hospital in London when I was being pushed through the corridors in the wheelchair. Christ knew what the pain was like and now I realised he understood the depression as well.

Next day I wrote, 'October 14th, 1982 Bad day physically, groggy all day but not one bit depressed.' At first I hoped it was an instant cure, but looking back through my diaries I can see I had to grope my way gradually out of that thick fog of depression with only occasional glimpses of 'light' to keep me going.

'November 1982 Can't do much, just hanging on and surviving. Life still seems very dark, but I know you're there now.' The most unexpected things seemed to help me during those months.

'December 1982 Tony took me and Naomi to see Kent Opera's *Fidelio*. When all those prisoners streamed out of their dark dungeon into the light of freedom the music was so lovely I suddenly remembered what joy feels like.'

'January 3rd, 1983 Found this quote today. It was scrawled on the wall of a Nazi cell in Cologne by a Jewish prisoner: "I believe in the sun, even when it's not shining, I believe in love even when I can't feel it, I believe in God, even when he is silent." I feel like adding, "I believe in happiness even when I can't feel it!"'

'February 15th, 1983   Grace took me for a lovely drive to Alfriston. We found a bank of snowdrops pushing their way out of the frost and ice. A promise?'

Looking back now I think one single event helped me more than anything else to kick that depression. It was probably May by then because the blossom was out all over the garden. It was such a fine morning. I was sitting out on the patio with a towel over my head to protect my eyes. Suddenly, energetic footsteps came running round the house, leaving me no time to hide.

'I've come to take you to the coffee morning,' said a friend brightly.

'Oh I don't think . . .' I began, coffee mornings have always been my pet aversion.

'It'll do you a power of good,' she insisted, and marched me in to change my dress. I was panicking badly but she did not appear to notice and drove me off to one of the largest houses in Mayfield.

The noise in the crowded drawing room was deafening as home-made jams and cakes were exchanged like priceless heirlooms. The chattering reminded me of an aviary full of budgies. Everyone looked so cheerful. As I shrank into a corner beside a mahogany bookcase I thought how well dressed and successful they all looked, standing in their little groups, toying with their shortbread biscuits. It was all very well for them, I thought. They had not had their lives destroyed, they could afford to 'chirrup' cheerfully away like that. (Surely self-pity is the ultimate disablement!)

There is one great disadvantage of living in a village. Everyone knows everything about you, but it works the other way too. You also know everything about them. As I looked from one to the other, I began to realise something. Behind those carefully applied masks nearly all those people were hurting too – perhaps continuously. Each had something which made life difficult. J with a broken marriage, M and her handicapped child, G who had built up a successful business with her husband only to see it crash catastrophically. Over in the corner was Mrs S whose husband had died after fifty years of marriage, and beside her sat T who had never married at all and lived with her senile mother.

My eyes continued to travel round the room searching for someone who lived an easy, happy life. I could not find one.

Here was I, complaining because my body was unreliable, but was that really any worse than living with a husband you couldn't trust? Wasn't loneliness a disability too? And what about grief and loss? Perhaps I had not been the only one singled out to play the lead in a tragic melodrama, the long slow secret griefs can hurt just as much as more dramatic ordeals. Trouble of one kind or another comes to all human beings sooner or later, so how had these people survived? Slowly it dawned on me that some of the kindest and most approachable people in the village community were here in this room. Their reaction to their problems seemed to have expanded them as people, while behind the masks of others were lines of resentment and bitterness. It occurred to me that while trouble is inevitable, growth is optional – and so is misery.

I went home feeling rather thoughtful.

'Thank you,' I said to my friend as we pulled up in front of our house.

'Told you it'd do you good,' she said. 'Takes you out of yourself doesn't it?' For once I did not find the cliché irritating.

It seems strange that I cannot find any reference in my diary to something which became as important to me as that coffee morning. At the time it obviously appeared insignificant, and it must have been more than two years before I thought about it again.

Chapter 8

Colour – glorious colour, that's what I remember most about the summer of 1983. The dismal gloom of the depression had finally dispersed leaving my world looking as if it had just been redecorated.

'It's only a rose Mum,' Justyn pointed out one day when he found me leaning on my stick and positively crying with joy.

'Yes, but just *look* at it!' I urged him. The physical problems were still there (for instance I still could not smell the rose), but I was learning to cope with them better. The pain had subsided to a dull ache and I was definitely stronger. The doctor at Burrswood had mentioned 'eighteen months' and for some reason I clung to that. Hope seemed to rise like sap. 'In six months' time I'll be completely well again,' I told myself. 'It was probably only the depression which made me give up hope.'

'July 1983   Went back to the WI again. *Such fun!*' If my friend had not forced me along to the coffee morning I would never have managed that. Once I had realised most other people felt vulnerable too, I was no longer shy of them and I stopped locking the door against callers. Soon it even became easy to lift the phone and say, 'Why not come down for a coffee?'

'The house is full of people again,' remarked one of the children that summer. 'It's just like the old days.'

The main source of my happiness was simply having something to do again. One day I was sitting under the apple tree telling the younger ones a story when Sarah came and leant over the back of the garden seat.

After we finished with the necessary, 'and they all lived happily ever after', she said, 'Mum, why don't you write a proper book? You always said you wanted to do that.' She was right, but the very idea made me smile ruefully. Great-auntie had dismissed the other part of my 'dream' because I could not spell. Dyslexia was my problem, but when I was at school teachers had never heard of the word. They had labelled me 'backward' instead. Covered in shame I would sit at the back of the class, wondering why everyone else could read and write, except me.

At thirteen I was still struggling to decipher the simple little books designed for five-year-olds. Yet I loved words, and used to play about with them in my head, listening to their rhythm as I strung them into sentences. My mother understood my frustration. She loved words too and wrote thirty-five books herself, but still found time to read aloud to me constantly. She knew what it felt like to have a mind which constantly teemed with stories and imaginary characters. So she encouraged me to dictate stories and, with the help of her secretary, I had even had a children's book published in the early 'sixties.

Learning to type helped my spelling slightly and eventually I did learn to read. My school-days may have ended in total failure, but story-telling was certainly an asset to the mother of a large family. Boring car journeys or long walks to the shops were never a problem. In the end, the need to write these stories down had become so great that I had banged them out myself on an old typewriter in the attic. Tony had to correct every other word with his red, teacher's pencil, but with his help I had finally published two more little children's books.

'Write a proper novel for people of my age,' Sarah's voice jerked me back to the scene under the apple tree. 'I'll help you.' I laughed at the idea of attempting to write a full-length book when I could not even spell words like 'becorse', 'enuff' or 'frend.'

'And besides,' I protested, 'I'm still not well enough to sit up at a typewriter yet.'

'You could if I made you a special table which fitted over your knees,' said Tony from his near-by potato patch. 'If your head and elbows were supported in a comfortable arm-chair, you'd be fine.' (My fingers at that time were still strong enough to press down the keys of an ordinary typewriter.) Throwing down his spade, he hurried away, and loud sawing noises and hammerings could soon be heard coming from his workshop. He loves making things, decorating the house, building furniture or designing toys for the children. He knew I had the same need to create and he had the sense to realise that if I could not ice a cake or embroider a tablecloth, then I must find some other way to express myself.

So the next morning, feeling a bit of a fool, I typed 'chaptor wun' at the top of a piece of paper and the hours the children spent at school never seemed to drag after that.

It was a perfect autumn that year and the trees seemed to blaze with colour. If inspiration flagged, we used to drive out into the woods and I worked sitting comfortably in the car.

By the end of October the manuscript was finished, and because Tony was obviously too busy to check my spellings we sent it to someone who advertised 'help with typing'. She told me spelling was her strong point, but six weeks later she rang to say she was on tranquillisers!

'You've made me lose my nerve,' she complained. 'I'm even having to look up words like *was* in the dictionary now.'

All the same, she did a grand job, and when Naomi had wrapped the manuscript up in brown paper, Sarah took it up to the post office one Saturday morning, addressed to a publisher. A few days later they sent back a slip saying, 'Your book will be dealt with in due course.' Although I watched hopefully for every post, we never heard another thing from them for more than a year, but at least they had not sent it straight back.

One frosty October evening I remember standing at my bedroom window. The apple tree looked so lovely in the moonlight.

'Everything's going to be all right again after all,' I thought. 'Even if the very worst happens and I never get much better than I am now, I still have everything in life I ever wanted. I can lie in bed at night and hear a fox barking across the fields, or look out of this window on a frosty morning and watch the sun rise behind the church steeple. Maybe one day they'll even publish my book.'

It was one of those 'flashes' of happiness, like the one when I went blackberrying in September 1981, but it was the last one I had for a very long time. It was only a few days after that when the entire family went down with colds. Massive doses of orange juice and fresh air soon righted them, but for me it was different. The mild infection triggered off a flare-up of the inflammation. It was not a serious attack and I did not even have to go into hospital, but suddenly all the pain and vertigo were back. It was exasperating when the fatigue and muscular weakness reduced me to crawling round like a great-great-grandmother once again. They say that banging your head against a wall makes it so nice when you stop. When you start again it feels twice as bad because you know how much it is going to hurt!

The consultant at the Kent and Sussex sent us back to the neurologist who had seen me in London. He ordered a whole range of electrical tests. Electrodes were stuck all over my scalp and other parts of my body.

'I was getting better, what went wrong?' I asked him later. He explained that I now appeared to have more than one problem. The first was the permanent damage left by the encephalitis. This showed up quite clearly in the tests as central damage caused when the nerves had been inflamed. He believed the scarring of the nerve casings meant it was taking

82

longer for the brain to send messages to other parts of the body. He also thought that some of my symptoms, particularly the constant pain and muscular fatigue, were because the inflammation of the brain and spinal cord had become chronic.* Perhaps it was just as well that he did not know that every time I came into contact with any kind of infection, such as a cold or flu, it could trigger off another major attack of acute illness. Four of these were just as serious, prolonged and life-threatening as the encephalitis in 1982 which I have already described.

'The more you rest,' he told me, 'and take life gently the fewer relapses you will have.'

'But there *must* be something more you can do.'

'I'm afraid there is actually nothing we can do, except treat the symptoms,' he explained gently. 'We can help to control the pain, inflammation and muscular spasms with drugs but there is no cure. You are just going to have to learn to live within your limitations from now on. Enjoy the good patches, Mrs Larcombe.'

Tony once described our lives from then on as a constant struggle to climb up from a deep coal mine inch by inch, then just before reaching the top, falling all the way back down again. My condition would improve gradually like it had that summer, and I would regain a modicum of mobility and independence. Then an infection would send me back into hospital again. Each time I had to start at the bottom once more as I faced months of rest, physiotherapy and dependence on other people. These attacks of encephalitis left me progressively weaker and more disabled. In between, there were less serious flare-ups and the myalgic encephalomyelitis caused continuous pain in head, neck and spine, muscular weakness and fatigue.

* Myalgic encephalomyelitis. A chronic inflammation of the brain, spinal cord, nerves and muscles. The condition can cause permanent damage to the central nervous system in some patients and also causes muscular weakness, loss of energy and poor general health. There is no known cure.

I often wonder if conditions which remain static – however disabling – are not actually easier to live with than things like multiple sclerosis (MS) and my kind of syndrome, which are constantly changing. For me the difference between a good patch and a bad one was enormous, and the uncertainties and variations in my abilities made life very unpredictable for the whole family. Sometimes I was on complete bed rest and needed a lot of nursing, while at others I was able to bath and dress myself. I could stagger about the house and do a few of the lighter jobs and even prepare simple meals. In spite of doing all those things at a snail's pace, they still boosted my morale. Even during the very best patches of all, however, I was not able to move easily, nor was I ever completely free of pain.

It was the patches of acute illness which Tony found particularly hard. While I was usually unaware of what was happening as I lay in the intensive care unit, he always knew my life was in danger.

For some time after we left the neurologist's consulting room I felt completely numb. Tony, on the other hand, saw clearly that the specialist's words spelt the end of our dream. While there was still hope I might recover, he had been willing to carry on alone with the mountainous chores involved in a country life-style. He had even managed to maintain the children's varied interests, which involved hours of driving them about both before and after his work each day. The strain of living like that was tremendous so, when the neurologist offered no hope of an end to the pressure, he began to feel that survival was more important than a dream. He decided we must leave our home in the country.

For a while he did not tell me how he felt; perhaps he knew just how devastated I would be by the thought of moving. Instead he became silent and morose, which baffled me completely. It is terrible to think how blind I was to his needs.

The significance of the visit to the neurologist dawned on me much more gradually, but at last I realised that, for me, time had not been the great healer – and neither had the medical profession. Accepting that something had devastated my life permanently was very difficult. Like most other people, I clung to the hope that there must still be some way out. A new pair of glasses had made reading for short periods much easier, so I began devouring books on Christian healing. It all seemed so simple. The books I read told stories of people recovering from all kinds of things after prayer, even advanced stages of cancer and the more I read, the higher my hopes soared. God loved us, so he would never allow our lives to be ruined like this.

One grey afternoon Tony took us all down to the seaside and while the children explored a ruined castle he and I sat on a seat in the icy wind.

'I can't go on any more,' he said suddenly.

'Whatever do you mean?' I asked.

'I just can't go on living in the country; it's all too much,' he replied dully. 'If we moved into Tunbridge Wells I'd be near the office. We must find a house without a garden, and if we lived close to the station and shops the children could be independent – take themselves where they need to go instead of me being a permanent chauffeur.'

'Live in a town? Near a station?' I repeated incredulously. To me the country was not just a pretty setting; beauty and tranquillity were as important to my spirit as food and drink to my body. We had twice tried living in a town and each time within months the most important part of me had begun to shrivel and dry up.

'You can't do this to me,' I said hoarsely. 'I can't survive without the woods and fields.'

'But you can't get out into them any more,' he pointed out. 'All the old things you used to enjoy are no good to you now; you've got to substitute new things instead, can't you see that?'

'I don't want a new life,' I said. 'I just want the old one back.'

'But you can't have it back, you've got to let it go.' He knew the idyll we had created so carefully was destroyed for us now. If we stayed hiding in its ruins it would become our prison: the only hope of happiness we had was to move on and build something new.

'Can't we just wait a little bit longer,' I pleaded. 'I feel sure God will heal me. I'll start going to Burrswood again – and other healing centres too.'

'You thought you were getting better last summer,' replied Tony wearily, 'but you can do far less now than you could then.'

'Well, if you're saying I'm going to be permanently disabled, then surely you must know I'll need the support of all my friends in the village more than ever.'

'You'll find loads of new friends in Tunbridge Wells.'

'No one would want to know a disabled woman,' I replied. 'I only have an identity here because they remember me as I was once.'

'Well you'll soon meet other disabled people.' I looked at him in sheer horror. Did he really think I wanted to be friends with people like Ellen, the woman in the next bed to mine in the Kent and Sussex? At that time I was still denying my long-term disabilities so firmly that even the sight of a wheelchair disturbed me profoundly.

'It wouldn't be fair on the children – forcing them to live in a town,' I said in an attempt to change the subject. 'And they're insecure enough as it is, without having to face new schools.'

'A change might help them,' muttered Tony, and his mouth had a mulish set – the point at which I knew argument was no longer worthwhile. We both retreated into silence while the cold wind whipped round us.

'Ninety per cent of marriages fail when one partner becomes disabled,' Madge had told me that, sitting in her wheelchair on the terrace at Burrswood. Her words still haunted me. Suppose Tony had been quiet and withdrawn recently because he was thinking of leaving me? Was he planning to sell the house so we could divide our resources? The thought was terrible, but why shouldn't he? My illness had certainly had a devastating effect on our marriage. Somehow I felt I had cheated him – I was no longer the kind of woman he had married. I loathed my new body and all its malfunctions and assumed he must feel the same way about it. Not being able to do things for myself had sapped my confidence and changed my personality. Now I was back in a bad patch silly little things had begun to worry me again. Dust on the dresser and shopping lists agitated me and instead of leaping out of bed in the morning full of zest and plans for the day, I was reduced to wondering how I was going to get my tights on.

The crippling fatigue and the pain not only interfered with physical contact but the constant effort of hiding it made me very vulnerable emotionally. When you dislocate a shoulder or slip a disc everyone expects the pain to make you 'touchy', but it is hard for them to go on making allowances when the pain persists indefinitely.

The children bounced up just then and interrupted our deafening silence by demanding ice-cream in spite of the cold. As Tony walked away with them towards the shop I wondered miserably how we would manage if he left us. Suppose he took them too? That thought was even more horrible. I could never be like Madge – content with just their photographs. If I was going to have to choose between my family and the country, then naturally they were what I wanted most. I would just have to suppress my opposition to this move if I was going to have any hope of keeping us all together.

Chapter 9

It took six months for the sale of the house to go through, and that winter felt like the 'dark night of the soul' for both of us. We were each locked into separate worlds, full of misery we did not dare discuss.

For Tony, the prospect of becoming a full-time carer was proving hard to accept. He first faced it in the hospital waiting room when he took me to see the consultant. Looking round he noticed two distinct groups of people: those who were obviously there to see the doctor, and the relatives who accompanied them. There were little old ladies fussing over frail husbands and middle-aged daughters with their elderly parents, a young mum with a baby on her hip and a husband who sat beside her, a pale, silent ghost of the truck driver he had been before his stroke. Tony said nothing to me at the time, but he remembers thinking, 'This is my new identity group. This is where I'm supposed to fit from now on.' Taking on the care of someone who is going to be ill for a long time means giving up your freedom and all kinds of ordinary things which most people take for granted. 'Laying down your life' for someone else involves a degree of love and unselfishness which is not often recognised by the rest of the world. Tony is a very cautious person. He likes to think everything out from all angles and although I was wrong when I assumed he was planning to leave us, he needed time and space to consider the implications of his new role.

Obviously it would have been unfair to tell me how he was feeling. Neither could I share my private anguish with him because I felt he was wrenching the countryside away from me without giving providence a chance to intervene.

I never doubted that God could heal me. It would not be difficult for Him, and our dream would then be preserved, our marriage saved and the children's security restored. I thought that all I had to do was approach Him in the right way. There must be some kind of a secret formula; once I had discovered it, my desire for health would be granted. So I flung all my energy into a search for a miracle. Many of my friends believed in healing, too, and together we prayed urgently and some of them even fasted. They lent me yet more books and cassettes on healing and offered suggestions and advice. 'Take zinc in large doses . . . switch to goat's milk . . . don't drink tap water . . . start deep-breathing exercises . . . try taking extra-strong vitamin pills.' They also told me about people who had recovered from all kinds of illness, and I listened hungrily, trying to discover how they had 'got it right'. Someone was always willing to transport me to services, healing centres or to visit people who were specially gifted. The quest was quite exhausting, but I felt I was working against the clock. It would be unthinkable to get better *after* we had moved to town.

On St Valentine's Day my friend Grace, a house mistress at the Mayfield Convent, dropped in to see me during her lunch hour. She found me huddled on the sofa in floods of tears. That morning I had written in my diary,

'February 14th, 1984   The only prayer I can utter today is *Help me*! Do something! It's half term but not for Tony so how do I entertain them all? Can't drive, can't walk. They're all out of hand, running wild. If you won't make me well, you might at least help me to be a bit better tempered!'

'Why doesn't God ever seem to answer my prayers?' I sobbed. She sat down beside me and did what, for Grace, was a very unusual thing – she began to talk. We must have been friends for at least six years by that time, but she is such a private person she had never told me before how she really felt when her husband had left her with four small children.

'I missed him badly, because I loved him so much,' she told me as she plied me with paper tissues. 'I was convinced that if I prayed hard enough God would mend our relationship and bring him back. So I positively wrestled in prayer – I even used to shout at God sometimes when the house was empty. In the end I was quite worn out, but still no husband. Then one day I found a tiny phrase in a poem written by Amy Carmichael [an author who was an invalid for many years]: "In acceptance lieth peace." I realised I had been demanding that God change my circumstances instead of looking for him in the middle of them. Acceptance was my watershed I suppose – it certainly led to peace.'

'But Grace,' I protested, 'acceptance is just a cop out. We must fight bad situations or they drown us.' She smiled her funny crooked smile at me and answered,

'When the Atlantic waves are rolling towards us they will drown us if we just weakly let ourselves sink under them – that's resignation. But acceptance is a strong act of the will, it means flinging ourselves on to the crest of the wave and allowing it to carry us into the shore.'

But I did not want to accept my life the way it was, and there were plenty of other people who were willing to offer me advice I liked better than Grace's.

'You must go to the Reverend X, he's got such a gift of healing,' one person told me. Someone else suggested a different healing centre altogether. Whenever I knew I was going to be prayed for, a great feeling of rising excitement would engulf me for days beforehand. This time it was going to work, and I would set off with my friends, convinced I would be well by the time I arrived home. The disappointment afterwards left me disillusioned and staggering under a load of despair. Soon Tony became thoroughly sick of it all.

'Why do you keep on putting yourself through all this?' he demanded in exasperation. 'Don't you realise it's tiring you out and making you ill, not better?' Each time I promised I would not allow my hopes to be raised again. Then someone else would come along with a new idea. I always felt I must try just once more, in case this time was 'it'.

During all those months I have to admit my relationship with God was not particularly comfortable. I only felt I could be useful to him and acceptable to other people if I was well. Health was a sign of God's approval, and illness still seemed like a total failure. The fact that he did not appear to be healing me in spite of all my efforts began to worry me greatly. Why? was the question which haunted me continuously. Perhaps I had offended God in some way, my faith was not pure enough or I had done something wrong. 'Please tell me what it is' I prayed earnestly. An overwhelming number of things came to mind: grudges, resentments, relationships that needed mending. Still, after confession and repentance, I was not healed. I found I was now fighting for my faith as well. If God was not going to do this one thing for me, then why should I go on with the farce of churchgoing and religious observance?

It positively infuriated me that Tony seemed to have reached that place of acceptance which Grace had told me about. One day when I was particularly irritated by his calm, I stood looking at the garden after the children had gone to school. It was a bright crisp day and all the trees and hedges were frosted white and sparkling like sugar in the sunshine. Even the dead leaves and twigs had become things of infinite beauty. Looking around at it all I found myself crying out to God in frustration. Later I wrote down what I had said in my diary.

'February 1984   Why are you letting all this be taken away from me? . . . Don't you realise all this loveliness *is* you to me, not just your creation, but a see-able feel-able *you*? I won't be able to worship you without it.' As I wrote I had the strange impression that words were forming themselves in my head. They seemed like some kind of an answer and I wrote them down underneath.

'I made all these beautiful things for you to enjoy, but now you must learn to see me in people not lonely beauty. In the old, sick and lonely, the depressed and tired. Love them just as you love those frosted branches.' For a while that helped me to be more positive, then I thought, 'That can't be a message from God; if he created us with a love for the country he would hardly send us to live in a town.' Tony's assertion that God could still love us and yet allow our lives to change was both unacceptable and irritating to me.

One day in March my frustration finally boiled over. I was standing with my nose pressed against the kitchen window looking longingly down the field towards the woods. In a few weeks' time that view would be replaced by streets, pavements and other people's cars. Suddenly it dawned on me that I would never see the blossom on the apple tree again. I had counted on something preventing the sale of the house, but now all the transactions were going through smoothly. My time had finally run out.

Behind me Tony rustled the *Daily Telegraph* contentedly as he read the sports pages over his breakfast.

'It'll be good when we get to town,' he said brightly. 'So easy for shopping.' For me *nothing* seemed good about living in Tunbridge Wells and as I turned away from the window all my suppressed anger erupted violently.

'I thought our life out here was important to you too,' I raged. Feeling both betrayed and abandoned, I picked up the steam iron in both hands and lunged it at where he sat. It missed his head and fell to the floor where it split open pathetically.

'Oh dear dear,' said Tony mildly without looking up from the paper. 'It's going to take at least fifteen pounds to buy a new one.'

Usually I talk far too much about the little things which do not really matter. Major things, however, seem to stick somewhere inside me. They didn't that day! Out they gushed as if from a breached dam and it was just as well the children were all out of earshot. I was astounded at the ferocity of my own vocabulary but suddenly I stopped in mid sentence. Tony was hunched over the kitchen table clutching his chest and his face was the colour and texture of putty. After a lot of coaxing he admitted he had been suffering from chest pains for some time. All my churning and resentment had done this to him, I felt sure of that, and I was positively frantic with guilt. For some reason that made me all the more angry with him.

'Why didn't you go to the doctor? It's just like your selfishness to go and die on me at a time like this!' He promised meekly that he would make an appointment at the surgery on Monday and went off to fiddle about with the carcass of the iron.

My head was so full of conflicting thoughts and feelings, I knew I had to be alone somewhere to think. I must get out into my blackberry field, just one more time. So when no one was there to say, 'Sit down, Mum, and stop being silly,' I shuffled my way across the garden on my two sticks, followed by Minty, our Jack Russell. At the bottom of our garden was a row of willow trees which hung over into the field beyond and provided a grand shelter for the cows. As I wriggled through the gap in the hedge I realised with some dismay that it had been raining hard for the last few days. While the cows had been gazing absently into space they had churned up the mud with their hoofs and done a lot of other unpleasant things as well. It was fortunate that I had lost my sense of smell.

Confronting me was a stinking mass of mud and dung which I would have to cross if I wanted to proceed on my excursion. Undaunted I felt with my sticks for the old railway sleepers which had always formed a path across the bog. It is far from easy to walk a plank when you have no balance and little control over your wellington boots, but I managed marvellously – until I was right in the very middle. The next sleeper wasn't there. I prodded anxiously with my stick as I felt myself begin to sink lower and lower in the mud and soon 'unspeakable unpleasantness' began to pour over the top of my boots. The more I floundered about the more trapped I became, and then slowly I keeled over, face downwards in what I described furiously as 'shit'. I gave up then and just sat there as the tears poured down my muddy face. Somehow the stinking filth seemed to be symbolic: it represented all the horrid things which had happened during the last two years. The more I struggled to get out of the mud, the deeper I sank into it, and it seemed to be the same with the problems.

'This is just like my life is now,' I told God furiously. 'Just a squelchy mess and I'm stuck in the middle of it.'

As I lay there beside myself with anger and frustration I believe God actually answered me. I didn't hear a voice or see a vision, but I felt without any doubt that He wanted me to know that he cared intensely about the mess. He was in the middle of it all with me, or He would be if only I would stop pushing Him away.

At first I was completely astonished. *Had* I been pushing him away? For months I had been convinced He had withdrawn his love from me because I had offended Him, could it really have been *me* who was offended with Him? Had my praying become a way of manipulating Him into doing what I wanted – making my own desires into my god? Wiping some more mud from my eyes I began to hand over all the things which were worrying me. Somehow they felt like the broken pieces of our carefully constructed dream: Tony's chest pains, my impaired body, the children's insecurity, the loss of our home and the threatening new life in town – everything. I asked God to take them all, and build out of them whatever He liked.

For months I had dreaded the day we would have to follow the removal van up the winding lane, but when the time actually came I did not need the wad of paper hankies I had stuffed up the sleeve of my jumper. Something had definitely happened to change me and I managed to cope with the move very well indeed. In that muddy bog I think I went through my barrier of acceptance. Grace had described acceptance as her watershed, and looking back now I can see it was the same for me. Perhaps peace comes when we stop asking the

94

question 'why?' and ask 'how?' instead. Not *why* did this happen to me, but *how* can I make the most of what I have left?

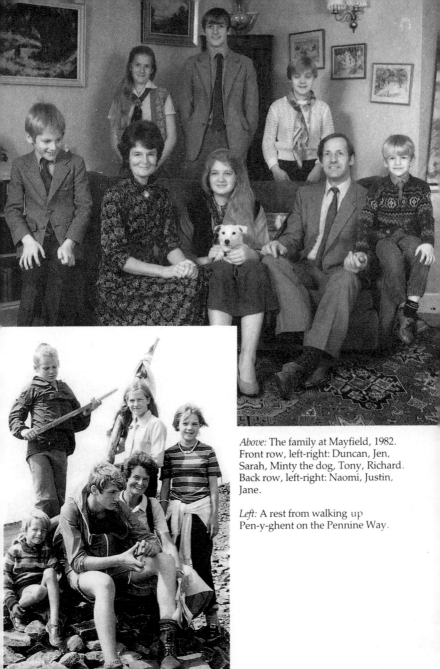

Above: The family at Mayfield, 1982.
Front row, left-right: Duncan, Jen,
Sarah, Minty the dog, Tony, Richard.
Back row, left-right: Naomi, Justin,
Jane.

Left: A rest from walking up
Pen-y-ghent on the Pennine Way.

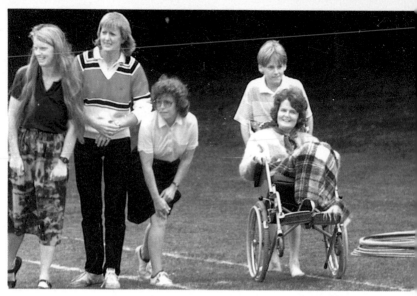

Above: The unforgettable Mothers' Race at the School Sports Day 1985. Duncan gets ready to push.

Below: 1986: left-right: Justin, Sarah, Duncan, Naomi, Tony, Jen, Minty, Jane, Richard.

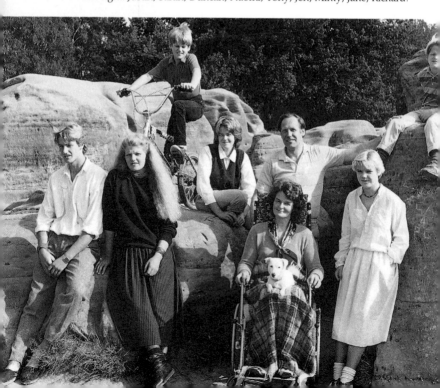

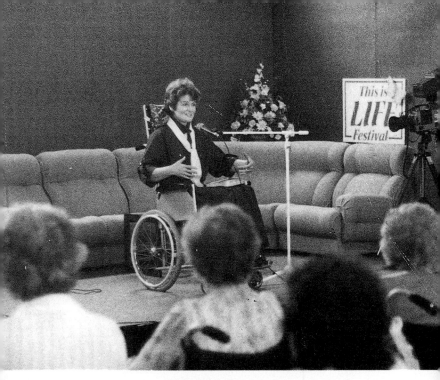

Above: A chance to speak to a group of disabled people in Bristol.

Below: Many hours were spent propped up in front of the typewriter.

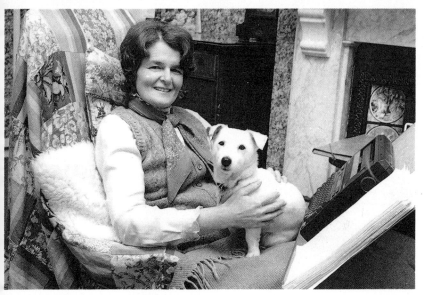

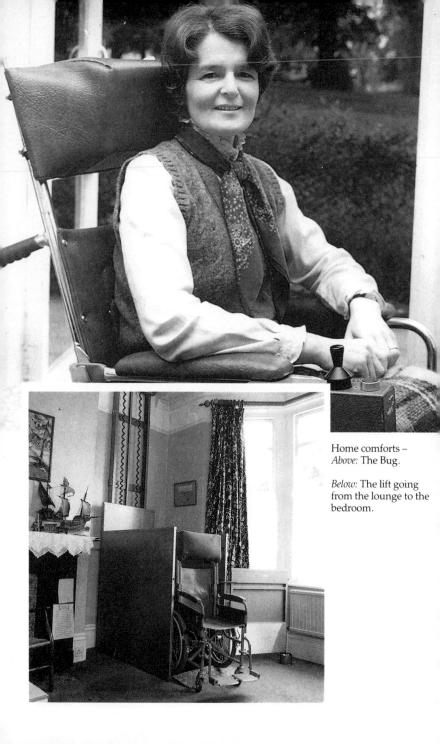

Home comforts –
Above: The Bug.

Below: The lift going
from the lounge to the
bedroom.

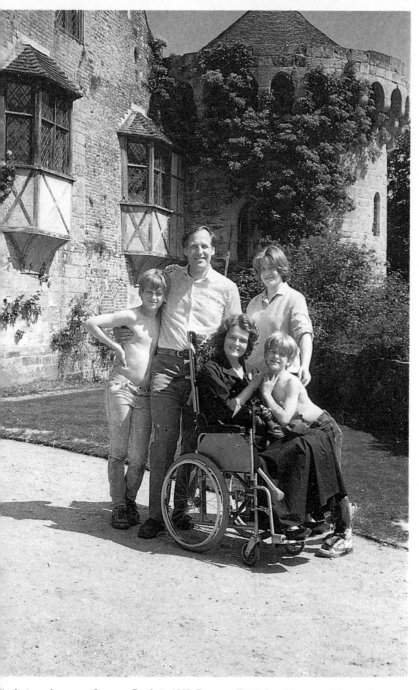

A glorious day out at Scotney Castle in 1987: Duncan, Tony, Jen, Naomi and Richard.

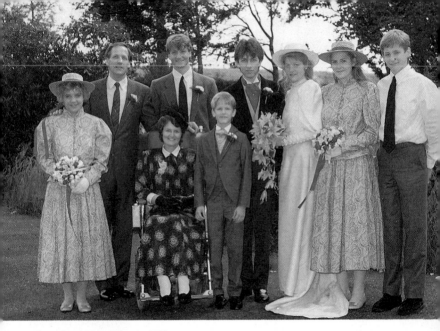

Above: Sarah's wedding in 1988.
Left-right: Jane, Tony, Jen, Justin, Richard, Paul, Sarah, Naomi and Duncan.

Below: Lyn checks up on Jen at the reception.

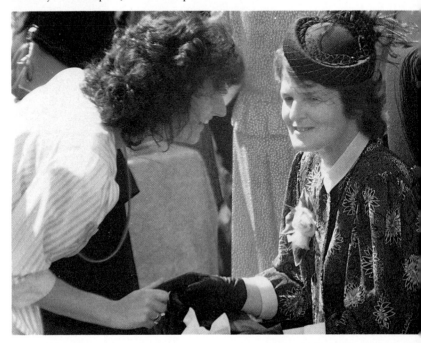

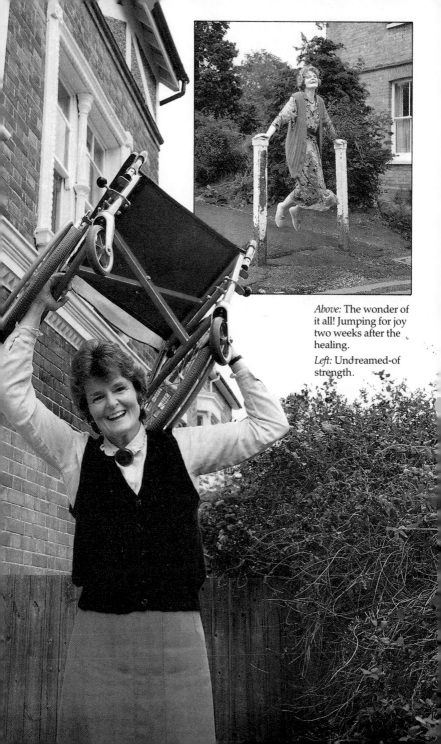

Above: The wonder of it all! Jumping for joy two weeks after the healing.

Left: Undreamed-of strength.

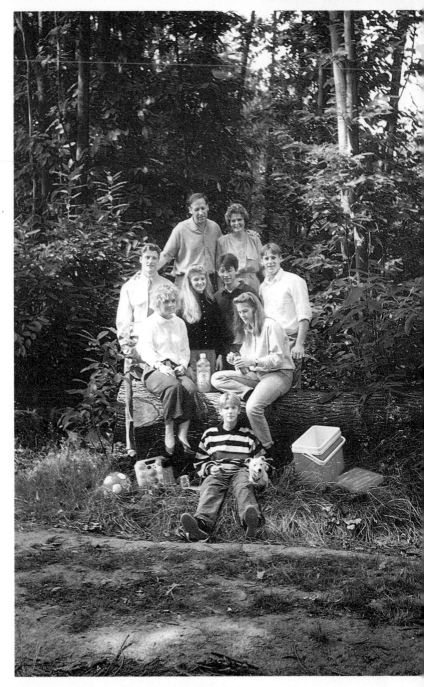

Glorious summer: a family picnic in August 1990.

PART TWO

Chapter 10

It was slightly annoying to discover Tony had been right after all. The benefits of the move became apparent right from the very first day and I was soon having to eat humble pie. The new house was an airy Victorian villa, large enough for the children to have a room each. It stood at the end of a terrace, and the big sash windows faced in three directions. From the kitchen we saw a yard where the dustbins stood and the dismal back side of the next terrace. The front of the house gave on to a street, but the side windows were my salvation. They looked out over the park. It was not one of those formal affairs, with symmetrical paths and flowers all standing at attention in neatly weeded beds. It was a wide expanse of green grass, dotted about with great shady trees. For me it was love at first sight, and I never grow tired of that view.

The other end of the street was not so much to my liking. It led into a main road and the shops, but the children thought being sent out to buy fish and chips for supper was the height of bliss. They all settled happily into their new schools and the street and park were a huge asset for skate boarding. We had wanted to create a perfect country environment in which to bring them up, but they loved being able to get about on foot or bus without having to depend on lifts. Obviously their freedom and friends were far more important to them than fields full of cows and blackberries. They even discovered that vegetables from the supermarket come ready scrubbed and slug free! Jane was particularly happy to be back in a town. She had spent her first seven years in Tunbridge Wells and the streets and shops felt like home to her.

One day, soon after we moved in, Tony was standing at the window, smiling.

'Just look at that!' he said happily pointing to the council gardeners cutting the grass in the park. 'There but for the grace of God go I!' Obviously much of his work load was lifted the moment we arrived in town, and seeing me become more peaceful also helped him to relax. Many of the tensions in our marriage were eased and soon I noticed he was looking years younger. The tests at the hospital had shown his chest pains were caused by stress, and now that his life was manageable he never complained of them again.

We had only been in Tunbridge Wells for a week or so when I decided to venture out alone to the post office. It was Tuesday, the day Child Benefit payments were made, and when you have six children it amounts to a nice juicy sum! To me, collecting the weekly allowance had always seemed part of motherhood. Now the post office was only round the corner, surely I could go and get it myself? Perhaps I would get to know some of the 'locals' at the same time. If ever you were lonely in Mayfield you only had to go to the post office to make friends; buying a single stamp could often take an hour and a half.

It was a glorious May morning when I set off, feeling as daring as if I was planning a solo crossing of the Atlantic. As a matter of fact, the pavement *did* heave about rather like the waves of the sea, but I was used to the sensation by then. I still walked leaning well forward for balance, my bottom stuck out like a duck. With my head held up firmly by a stiff surgical collar, I managed to shuffle along the pavement with my two sticks. With both hands occupied, a handbag was always a problem, so I hung it round my neck where it dangled like a horse's nose-bag. Even with my darker than dark glasses I could hardly have looked like a film star, but at least I felt I was achieving something.

By the time I reached the corner I was already so tired I

wished I'd stayed at home. The traffic seemed to hurtle in all directions, trains rattled into the station at the bottom of the hill and the tall Victorian buildings towered above me like prison walls. 'I should have gone in the park instead,' I told myself nervously, but I hated giving up. Negotiating the pedestrian crossing came next. I shuffled over the road as fast as I could, but a young man in a sporty red car blasted his horn and shouted morale-denting comments about old age pensioners.

When I finally staggered up the steps of the post office I was sweating with exhaustion, but there wasn't a chair in sight. The place was positively bulging with people that day and only one harassed man peered at us through the wall of glass. Standing in the queue was difficult. I was never quite sure where my head was in space so I had to concentrate like mad to keep myself upright. It felt like fighting a constant battle with my own muscles. When the line moved forward I found I could not make my legs work fast enough to keep up.

Everyone else seemed to be in a furious hurry and I became aware of the irritation my slowness was causing when the opulent lady behind me started to sigh loudly. Perhaps that was the first day I realised that as a disabled person I was no longer welcome in crowded places. If anyone doubts me let them try going to Woolworths in a wheelchair a week before Christmas.

By the time I finally reached my turn at the counter, the large lady's sighs had turned into indignant tut-tutting. When you need two sticks to keep you upright, scrabbling round in your handbag for your allowance book is a complicated procedure. The tutting was catching and the tension in the queue behind me mounted as I fumbled to separate the pages. I felt like a freak under the hostile glare of so many pairs of eyes. Signing my name was always a laborious business and when I dropped my purse and shot coins in all directions the large lady behind me positively snorted. Then the worst happened. I had leant my heavy-headed National Health walking sticks against the counter, but they slowly began to slide sideways and crashed down on to the snorter's foot. She was wearing open-toed sandals! The dance of the sugar plum fairy is hardly a good description of her furious capering. If only I could have run away, but my exit was maddeningly slow.

When at last I managed to get myself down the steps I leant against the wall at the bottom and closed my eyes against the whizzing cars and swirling pedestrians. Never have I felt so embarrassed or more disabled. 'I don't want to live in this town,' I thought. 'And I don't want to look like a freak.'

The human memory is an extraordinary device. Why, at a moment like that should I think of an irritating remark my father always made at moments of family crisis? If I fell off my bike, lost my best friend or ripped my party dress, he would always say, 'Never mind, the Good Lord knows what He's a-doin' of.' At that moment the words seemed to fill my entire mind. Yes, I thought, with a sudden feeling of reverence. He *does* know what He's a-doin' of. This illness was not a failure, a mistake or a punishment. God had allowed it for a reason we did not yet understand. He had taken all those broken pieces of our lives when I gave them to Him in the muddy bog, and He knew what He was going to build with them.

Ever since that Tuesday, I have never been able to go past the post office without remembering what happened next. It was another of those 'flashes' of happiness, like the time I went blackberrying or looked out of the window at the moonlight. The circumstances could not have been more different or less pleasant, but the happiness was the same. It poured right through me.

That day I learnt happiness actually has nothing to do with outside happenings. The next few years were far from easy for any of us in the family, but we began to have this solid inner contentment which only someone who has experienced it can possibly understand. We later christened it our 'peace-joy'.

As I crawled slowly towards home that day I found I was thinking about Great-auntie and her high ideals. Well, now I would never achieve the kind of things she would have approved. I would never be a Florence Nightingale or a Mother Teresa. But if God had allowed me to be a disabled person, then surely I could expect Him to help me do it well, just as I would have done if He had given me some other vocation.

Somewhere about then I resolved never again to pray for healing. It was not that I stopped believing God could heal me, it was simply that I felt it was now His responsibility. Mine was to get on and enjoy life as much as I could. I felt I was making a very definite pledge when I wrote this in the back cover of my Bible:

'Spring 1984   I promise you Lord, I will never ask again (for healing) . . . Mend me if you wish or use me as I am . . . weak and sick. Let me leave the symptoms and pain in your sacred province and turn away from them now towards other people.'

It was some years before I discovered a writer called Rosanna Benzi, but she described exactly how I felt at that time. After an attack of polio she spent her adult life in an iron lung and wrote several books. In one – *The Vice of Living* – she says, 'I do not ask God to get me out of here, I trust him. I must say I think its mutual.'

There were several practical things which also contributed to our feeling of well-being. One was the support we received from our new doctor. To find a GP who shared our faith meant a lot to us all, but Tony particularly derived great confidence from his kindness and understanding, especially during the times when I was in hospital.

'You need a home help for at least two hours a day,' he told us the very first time we met. 'Leave that to me and I'll send the OTs round too. They can fix you up with rails, ramps and all kinds of gadgets to make life easier.'

To me, occupational therapists had something to do with basket-work and knitting, but I was wrong. When I could no longer climb the stairs, they installed a lift which propelled me through the lounge ceiling and deposited me and my wheelchair in the bedroom. I could never decide who was most pleased with it, me or the children! The OTs also arranged a device which made it possible for me to open the front door by touching a button by my chair. They produced tables on wheels, gadgets for the bath and special feeding utensils when they became necessary. But just for the record, they *did* also teach me how to weave cushion covers, and the satisfaction I gained from making something myself again was indescribable. One day recently I heard someone making a joke about the rush-seated stools made by disabled people and I nearly punched him.

To be honest, I was very apprehensive at the idea of the home help. I visualised a large, strong-minded woman thrusting her huge bust through our front door and usurping my role as a mother. So Lyn was a very pleasant surprise. She was small, pretty and wore a track suit. Over the next six years she became my hands and feet but left my dignity intact. Almost as soon as she arrived in July 1984 I began another flare-up which landed me in hospital in London for two months and then confined me to bed at home for several more. She became a substitute mum right from the start and during all the many times when I was away she created the security and stability the children had lacked when I had been ill before. During bad patches she had to do almost everything for me, and only a very exceptional kind of person can rebuild self-confidence in the patient who is so completely in their power. Perhaps Lyn managed it because she taught me how to laugh again while she washed me, helped me to the loo or did up my buttons. I used to store up all the funny things to tell her when she came in each morning and when you can laugh about falling over or wetting your pants, somehow it does not seem so humiliating. She had another important quality of a good carer. When the good patches came she let me have my independence back, even though it must have been frustrating. She would watch me making a cup of coffee or tidying a room – she could have done it so much faster herself but she still let me do it at my own pace.

She also coped with the complicated matter of my pills. By that time I was taking a vast amount each day. Three kinds of pain-killers, varying in strength. Muscle relaxants to control the spasms. Anti-inflammatory drugs. Pills to help the vertigo, another to prevent nausea and a good many more besides. I hated the thought of them all so much I never could be bothered to work out what I was supposed to take – and when. Not being able to remove the bottle tops was my excuse. So Lyn used to leave each day's supply ready in an idiot-proof plastic container with four sections. Without her to organise me, I would probably have got into a dangerous muddle.

During that first winter the neurologist in London and our own doctor felt I should be placed on the Disabled Person's Register. Before my walk to the post office I doubt if I could have coped with the finality of that. Yet we soon discovered how helpful this new status was. It made me eligible for all the various state benefits. The lengthy procedure involved in gaining the Attendance Allowance, Mobility and Severe Disability Allowance gave Lyn plenty of scope for humour. Three different NHS doctors had to come to the house and examine me at various times. That could have been very degrading had she not defused the unpleasantness of the situation by listening in and giving them marks out of ten for their bedside manner!

'I'm not sure I'm going to like being a drain on the state for the rest of my life,' I told Lyn doubtfully.

'It's a darn sight better than being a drain on Tony,' she replied briskly. She was right, of course, even though I felt receiving help was a bit embarrassing at first. Those weekly payments helped Tony in all kinds of ways. They paid for Michelle for one thing. It had been quite an undertaking for Tony to see that a meal was provided for eight people each day – not to mention all those school packed lunches. So it was a huge relief to him when Michelle arrived each afternoon and did all our cooking. As the children tucked into her chocolate pudding they always used to say,

'We're glad you're ill, Mum,' and Tony began to put on a little weight. So did I, which was just as well, seeing I had gone down to only six and a half stones. Weight Watchers had given me a goal weight of ten stones four pounds when I joined some years before. Jane used to giggle at the sight of my spindly legs and tell me I looked like a shrivelled-up monkey.

'Well it's better than paying out to go to Weight Watchers,' said Lyn defensively, but I did not mind because it was so good just to hear Jane laughing again.

When we first moved into the street I felt as if we were living in a goldfish bowl. Soon I discovered the fish confined in the bowl had an excellent view! All day long a constant stream of people flowed past the house and I could watch them from my bed or the reclining chair. My windows faced both the street and the park, and soon I began to recognise the various faces as they dashed to catch the London trains. I invented names for the young mums who pushed their prams towards the swings and I watched love affairs develop as office workers met for lunch under the trees. Sometimes on hot summer evenings the patrons of rival pubs engaged in noisy battles which were far more entertaining than the television. I became so involved in watching all these nameless people, the woods and fields I had seen from my windows in Mayfield seemed rather dull by comparison.

In the country we had lived round the kitchen table. Now that I had to spend much of my time lying down the whole family seemed to take up residence in my large bedroom. They all said they liked having a 'static' mother who was always there to play a game, read aloud or watch a television 'soap'. Minty liked having me in the same place all the time as well and she was very good company over the years.

My bedroom also became a substitute for our old garden. I lay surrounded by so many plants and vases of flowers that Lyn christened it 'Kew Gardens'. She nearly had a fit when

106

Naomi filled flowerpots with soil from the garden and worms escaped and crawled all over the pink carpet.

'Think what they'll do to my cleaner,' she complained. Her feelings were mild, however, in comparison to the horror of the district nurse when Naomi helped me plant up pots of bulbs all over the bed and the peat escaped and vibrated about in the ripple mattress she had just installed.

One day during our first winter in town, Lyn found me rather less cheerful than usual. It was soon after I had received the letter from the social security department telling me that I was now officially registered as a disabled person. Even though I knew my new status would help us, it was still a blow to the morale. Suddenly I was not sure that living life through my children and the bedroom window was going to be quite enough for me. Even Lyn's usual jokes did not lift my spirits.

Then the phone rang. A voice I did not recognise told me she was the senior editor of the publishing house where I had sent my teenage novel more than a year before. Their long silence had not bothered me because I never seriously expected them to like it — any more than my school teachers relished my homework.

'I've just read your manuscript. We've had a staff reshuffle here, that's why we've been so long in bringing it out.' Lyn told me later I sat there with my mouth open like an astonished toad. Was the voice telling me the book would be published? 'I'd like to come down and see you,' continued the editor. 'When would that be convenient?' There was no point in scanning my diary — all the pages were blank, but I wasn't going to tell her that.

'I do seem to be free around midday tomorrow,' I said with a gulp. 'Why don't you come for lunch?'

'Whatever do publishers eat?' asked Lyn suspiciously.

The following day seemed to take a long time to arrive. When Lyn finally ushered in my visitor and her huge bunch of flowers, she said with a sigh, 'They'll be holding Chelsea Flower Show in here soon.'

I remember thanking Christine, the editor, profusely for everything I could think of and saying I was sorry for everything else. Then I finally sank back into shyness. During two and a half years of illness I had developed what I call, 'the disabled mentality': you even say 'thank you' in your sleep and apologise for breathing. So I was astonished when she opened our conversation by saying, 'I've come to ask if you would like to write two more novels about the same characters – so we can make them a trilogy.'

'Thank you,' I said weakly. I was so surprised I had to struggle hard not to cry. Moments like that do not come very often in a lifetime. To give me a chance to recover, Christine went over to the window, 'What a lovely view you have of the park, it must be beautiful in summer.'

'Oh yes,' I said, 'and it's such fun watching all the different kids playing out there. In fact I was thinking of writing a children's book about them.'

'I'd like to publish that one as well,' said Christine promptly.

'Three books!' I thought jubilantly when she had gone. Later the phone rang again; this time it was the editor of a magazine called *Family* asking me to do a series of articles on child rearing. I was so excited I wanted to express my feelings by dancing round the room or leaping into the air. Instead I could only purr with satisfaction – but that did not matter. Now I was a real person again who actually 'did' something. If I ever had to fill in a form and answer the question 'occupation' I would not have to say, 'disabled person' or even 'housewife'. I could put 'writer' now.

There was one small problem, however. My fingers were no longer strong enough to use an ordinary typewriter. But even that difficulty was overcome when a friend who had just lost her husband sent a cheque through the post one morning. 'I felt you might be needing an electric typewriter,' she said. Tony went straight out and bought me a small portable machine with a very light touch. It fitted on a sloping table which could be pulled over my bed or the reclining chair.

Provided I was almost lying flat and my arms were well supported the pain was kept at bay and I could work without undue fatigue for quite long stretches.

After that I never found the days were long enough. First I wrote children's books. The stories used to 'happen' inside my head as if I was watching an internal video. It felt a bit like cheating really, because I needed help from the whole family. In the evenings the children would snuggle into my bed to hear the latest chapter and advise me about what should happen next. Then Tony had the unenviable task of correcting all the spellings.

Non-fiction books for adults came next. They were more of a challenge (but rewarding all the same). A different publisher, Hodder and Stoughton, commissioned the first one, and no one was more surprised than I was when it made their 1986 bestsellers' list. When their editor rang to ask if she could come and see me about another book to follow it up, I was most excited. Unfortunately the interview did not turn out quite as well as I hoped. Previously a different editor had worked with me, so I had never met this one before. Someone told me she was rather hesitant about commissioning a book because of my precarious health. So I desperately wanted to reassure her I could be trusted to meet a deadline. I decided not to see her in my bedroom, and pictured us talking downstairs in the lounge, with me sitting in an ordinary chair, my hair neatly set and an efficient-looking clipboard at the ready.

It was too bad that her arrival should have coincided with a bad pain day. Every day there was pain but usually, if I could settle down at my keyboard, the writing had the marvellous effect of diverting my attention. Bad pain days were different; they flattened me completely because I was sick so many times. Lyn used to draw my bedroom curtains and leave me alone. Not even her jokes worked when the headache was that bad. Some of the strong pain-killers I was sometimes prescribed, such as Palfium and MST (morphine sulphate slow release) caused me to be terribly sick. The district nurse used to come and give me injections of Stemetil to try and counteract this but often they had little effect.

It never occurred to any of us to put off my editor's visit. 'The show must go on' was a motto which really helped us as a family to cope with the illness. When Tony brought her upstairs, she must have thought it rather strange to be entertained in almost total darkness by someone who was flat on her back and vomited five times during the interview!

'Take no notice,' Tony told her casually. 'It often happens.' Lyn was always as unflappable as he was: she simply emptied the bowl without embarrassing me with sympathy. All the same, I noticed our visitor did not touch the nice little lunch Michelle had left her on a tray and it was more than a year before she said anything more about the next book.

Tony's endless patience over my spelling was remarkable but when that new book was finally under way even he began to grow a little weary. So did the typewriter. One day he came home with a gleam in his eye and a very large box.

'I'm confiscating your typewriter for a whole week,' he said firmly.

'You can't do that,' I said in alarm. 'I've got an article to finish.'

'You can have it back later – *if* you still really want it,' he said as he drew a computer out of the box.

'Oh no!' I groaned in horror. 'I hate those things!' During the ghastly week which followed, I waded through the handbook in confusion and despair. I pleaded for my typewriter often but just when Tony was about to relent, I suddenly realised what this monster could mean to me. I could play about with words and phrases without having to retype the whole page, change a paragraph into the past tense or move it right into another chapter, then delete it altogether if the idea failed to work. Best of all, I discovered the spelling check.

Ever since then the computer and I have been almost inseparable, and it is a good thing Tony bought one with a large memory, because there are an awful lot of books stored in there now. Sadly, his red pen is still needed because computer

110

technology is not yet advanced enough to know the difference between here and hear, there and their, or to, too and two!

The books were all fun to do, but I think I found writing for magazines and papers even more satisfying. Over the years I was asked to contribute regularly to ten of them. Some were aimed at parents, others were for women. One catered for disabled people, while the local paper wanted pieces giving the Christian angle on community affairs.

'There's an article in that,' I would say whenever something interesting or funny happened and that saying became a family joke.

The lovely thing about writing was that I could go on doing it during all the ups and downs of the illness. I could work in bed in the bad patches and in my reclining chair during the better ones.

One night Tony and I were watching an Australian television programme. I remember that particular episode vividly and I find I have described it in my diary, so it must have meant a great deal to me at the time.

'February 13th, 1987 Saw *Prisoner Cell Block H*. Old woman (who has been inside for so many years all the other prisoners rely on her for everything) was very worried when the time came for her release. Governor said, "You'll be fine, lots of people out there will help you." Old prisoner replied, "But you don't want to be helped, you want to be wanted."'
That last phrase is underlined heavily in my diary, and it would probably also be the cry of most disabled people who feel constantly on the receiving end. My greatest need was still to be able to give. A friend, Dave, is a sculptor, in spite of the fact he is blind. Jill is encased in a moulded plastic frame but she still paints exquisite landscapes. Margie does the same – by holding the brush in her teeth. Their work gives a great deal of pleasure to others. Although I wrote mostly because I adored doing so, whenever someone told me a book or an article of mine had made them laugh, or helped them see something from a new angle, I used to feel that my life, with all its restrictions was worthwhile after all.

111

Chapter 11

That inexplicable brand of inner happiness was not something we always found easy to maintain. There were certain occasions when we lost our 'Peace-joy', and family holidays were definitely one of them. The wheelchair (when I finally succumbed to one) took up a vast amount of room in the car, loos were never there when I needed one urgently and finding suitable accommodation was increasingly difficult. We would probably have taken all those things in our stride if we had not always made the mistake of going back to the 'old haunts' of my well days.

'August 26th, 1985   Everything reminds me of what we did before and the things I can't do this year.'

'August 23rd, 1986   Terrible day, children all pulling in different directions. It is quite impossible for Tony to go on a self-catering holiday with a handicapped person and six energetic children. I'm *so* exhausted and he's so bad tempered.' And he was! But then so was I. Our reasons were very different, however. My bad moods were usually caused by a serious illness known as POM (Poor Old Me). I seemed to develop an attack of it whenever we went away. We had always been the kind of family who like active holidays – fell walking, playing golf or exploring rocky coastlines. Suddenly none of those things was possible for me and I loathed being stuck in the car while the rest of the family disappeared up the side of a mountain.

For the first week of that holiday in 1986 we stayed in our favourite Quaker youth hostel in the Lake District. One day they all decided to climb Haycocks at the far end of Lake Ennerdale. As usual I was left behind in the noisy car park and when they seemed to be gone for an interminably long time, the 'POMs' began with a vengeance. Jealously I eyed other mothers pounding off up the mountains with knapsacks bobbing on their backs and even when it began to pour with rain, I still envied them their freedom. By the time my lot finally came into view I was positively spitting with rage.

'But Mum,' explained Naomi gently, 'we couldn't help being so long. Poor old Dad had an accident on the scree and he's cut his wrist open badly.' Even the pathetic sight of Tony hobbling round the corner – bloodstained and shaken – could not soften my bad temper.

'Serves him right,' I snapped. 'If I could still climb a mountain I wouldn't care if I cut my hand right off while I did so!' That, too, became a family joke – like throwing the iron.

Tony's bad temper was something I simply could not understand until recently. It was caused by guilt because he still *could* climb the mountains. The children had inherited our love of physical activity so he naturally needed to go with them on all their hair-raising adventures. He felt bad when he enjoyed himself, knowing how I hated being left behind. Every time they discovered a rare wild flower he wanted me to be there to enjoy it too. Yet he did not dare come bounding back to tell me all about it in case I bit his head off.

Without Lyn and all the labour-saving gadgets of home, it was much more difficult for us both to cope. We loved staying in the Quaker hostels because they were cheap and near the mountains – but unfortunately they were also extremely primitive. That particular year I was on a drug which made me very sick indeed and we missed the district nurse and her injections. We did not dare to go to a local doctor, however, in case he said we should not be staying in a damp youth hostel out in the wilds, and packed us all off home. We wanted to go on to a similar hostel in Yorkshire for the second week.

It was while we were staying there that something happened which helped me to regain my Peace-joy. One fine evening we went to Malham Cove, a huge limestone cliff with a river at the bottom which Kingsley used as a setting for his book *The Water Babies*.

Naturally they all wanted to climb to the top and after settling me in a deck-chair with plenty of insect repellent they set off. Soon they looked as small as gnats themselves as they zigzagged up the treacherous path.

'Why did you let this happen to me, Lord?' I prayed as the tears ran down my cheeks. 'Surely I could have done so much for you, if only I could have been healthy and active.'

It was just like the muddy bog. The answer was inaudible but totally clear. A writer never goes anywhere without a notebook so I jotted down what I felt I had heard.

'Many people work for me, but very few are willing to be my friends. That's what I want you to be. It's your company I desire more than anything. Learn to sit and look at things and enjoy them with me.' Ever since then that personal friendship with God has been the most important part of my life. If I had never been ill I might have bustled about doing all the admirable things Great-auntie would have wanted, but I could have missed something which has given me more delight than anything else. Of course He was offering me His friendship before, just as He does to everyone and anyone, but I would probably have been too busy to have realised that.

Once in hospital I met a girl called Jane who has become a close friend. All her life she has been dogged by bouts of illness and during one of them she said to me, 'When your need for God is paramount, that is when you really know him.' That certainly was my experience too.

The following day they all decided to climb Ingleborough. From the moment they left I knew I had my Peace-joy back. Just sitting and looking at the great purple hill was fascinating. The cloud shadow changed its colour so many times during the four hours they were gone.

'What is this life – if full of care, We have no time to stand and stare?' Those words had always annoyed me in the old active days, but after that holiday I began to make an art of 'just looking'. It would have astonished me to discover what a delight I could derive from an amaryllis bulb on my window-sill or the trees in the park blowing in the wind. Communicating with God was not always easy in words, but I used to feel that enjoying beautiful things with Him was a form of prayer. In Mayfield, whenever I wanted to pray, I found it easier if I went for a walk through the fields. Now I could no longer do that but I discovered music was a good substitute (when my ears were not being 'difficult'). Sometimes when I felt particularly 'imprisoned' by my painful body I used to put the cassette player on very softly and picture myself walking in a wood or on a mountainside. It sounds absolutely ridiculous, but to me then it was a huge release and I discovered it was perfectly possible for my mind and spirit to be free even if my body was trapped.

In spite of this beautiful new dimension to life, I have to confess that my peace was something which could evaporate very easily indeed: when I could not wrap a birthday present or decorate the Christmas tree, for instance.

Tony did not seem to have as much bother with it. His faith is stronger than mine and he has a more even temperament. There was really only one occasion when Peace-joy really deserted him, but unfortunately the experience lasted for six long months. It began after I had the fifth serious attack of encephalitis, in March 1987. That particular 'acute episode' seemed to get to him more than all the others. As usual it began very suddenly. One day I complained of a sore throat, the next I was too sleepy to be roused easily and the pain in my head and neck became severe. When Lyn heard me muttering about 'Baa baa black sheep' who needed a hankie, Tony knew it was time to ring the doctor. When I could no longer swallow he always had to have me admitted to hospital so that fluids could be administered intravenously. I also needed to be attached to a diamorphine pump (a very powerful drug normally given to terminal patients with severely painful conditions). I do not remember the ambulance ride which, Tony tells me, took place late at night, but he remembers it all far too well. He felt as if he was watching a horror video he had seen too many times already.

Over the next few days he spent hours sitting beside me in the intensive care unit while I lay there oblivious to his presence. He had seen it all before – the pump, drips, catheter, oxygen mask – and my body had become a part of their complex machinery once again. When a doctor explained that I was not expected to live more than a few more hours at the most, Tony believed him, even though that kind of thing had been said to him on other occasions. As he sat there beside me he felt that he had reached the very end of his own resources. He could find no more courage or will power left to carry him on. He decided this feeling probably indicated that this time he was going to lose me.

He is a very active man, and doing nothing is virtually impossible for him. So as he sat there beside the bed, he began to pray out loud, thanking God for all the things we had done together over the years. The life in Mayfield, the games of golf and the birth of each of the children. It took him a long time but it helped him greatly. When it was time to go back to the children, he said what he thought was his last goodbye and walked away home down the hill. He says the tears were spurting out horizontally, but something happened to him before he arrived. He will never talk about it except to say that he was comforted.

When he was told a few days later that I had survived yet again his reaction was not one of relief. He simply could not face having to go through the goodbyes all over again the next time I caught a cold. Nor could he stand the thought of watching yet another exhausting struggle up out of the coal mine which always followed an attack of encephalitis. He had simply had enough. It must be a ghastly experience walking right up to the edge of death with someone you love very much, but when you have to do it several times it becomes a torture you just cannot face again. He had to cope with the children's distress as well as his own, and he found himself thinking – if death has to come, then it would be far less strain on us all if it happened soon.

When I was finally allowed home he did not seem able to let himself enjoy my company. He continued to care for me physically but emotionally he withdrew – perhaps to protect himself from future pain. If only he could have told me how he was feeling, then I would not have felt so completely abandoned.

We went on existing in isolation like that until November. By then I was desperate and beginning to wonder once again if his silence meant he was thinking of leaving. So I persuaded him to go with me to visit our friends who are Christian counsellors in Southampton. Hugh and Ginny did not give us any advice – what could they possibly have said in a situation like that anyway? They simply encouraged us to talk and at last we each began to realise how the other was feeling. It had never dawned on me just how stressful it was for Tony to live in the present with someone, when he did not feel we shared a future. Naturally there was nothing I could do about it, but it helped so much to know that he had not withdrawn because he did not love me, but simply because he loved me too much.

If ever I had friends who were facing the approach of death I would always say, 'talk to each other about how you really feel'. It sounds very noble to say, 'I'm shielding him from worry', but in our experience, silence only increases the worry because it leaves too much to the imagination.

It makes me want to cry now, as I imagine how Tony must have felt that day in Southampton as he tried to struggle back again through the acceptance barrier to a place of peace. Those years of living in an uncertain limbo must have been so very much harder for him than for me. I don't know what really went on in his head that day, it is something he cannot put into words. What I do know is that our friends prayed for him a lot and when we drove home in the car he and I were close to each other again. We have stayed like that ever since.

During the journey we discussed practical coping strategies. It was obvious that he was going to need friendships and interests outside our home. The daily running of the household no longer revolved round him as it had in Mayfield. Lyn shouldered so much of the responsibility and, although Michelle had left us by then, Gom, my old nanny, came in most days. If all Tony's fulfilment continued to be centred on our life together then the devastation of losing me would be too great. Satisfaction was what he badly needed and he had to find that through his career and in the kind of hobbies and interests in which I could not join him. I had my writing, which provided my fulfilment. In a way I had to let him go emotionally, and he had to let me go as well. It sounds like a horrific conversation in cold blood, but we needed to talk all those things through and, strangely, it relieved the pressure in our relationship.

It was very important for Tony to have friends who valued him for himself and not just as 'poor Tony whose wife is so ill'. He found just that kind of acceptance and support in our Baptist church. So did the children, and I used to feel so safe knowing they all had people there who would support and care for them whatever happened to me. About that time Tony was asked to become an elder and take more of a lead in church affairs. In view of our discussion he felt it was something he should do. Although I did not have the energy to become as involved as he was, it provided us with a common interest which was very important.

During those six months when Tony was having such a struggle, many things were churning round in my mind too. In hospital during the previous March and April the doctors had talked about sending me home with a morphine pump

118

attached to my arm. They felt it would be a more consistent form of pain control than swallowing MST tablets. I was not too happy with the idea and said to a nurse, 'Aren't you worried that you'll turn me into a junkie?'

'We don't bother about things like that with terminal cases,' she replied with a smile. I insisted on going home without the pump. I was not going to die yet, whatever she thought. All the same the word 'terminal' left a nasty taste in my mouth.

During that summer I began writing a new book which involved a lot of research into the subject of suffering and a God of love. It was a very difficult book to write, particularly while my relationship with Tony was causing me so much misery. One day in late October, just before we went down to Southampton, some of the children took me out for an airing in the wheelchair. We were outside the local supermarket when we saw a woman leaving the shop with two bulging polythene bags of groceries. A yappy little dog ran between her legs and over she went, sprawling over the pavement. Her overstuffed bags burst open, exploding tins, oranges, bottles and eggs in all directions.

The chaos was indescribable but before any one could run to help she bounced up like a jack in the box and said brightly, 'Not to worry, I'm off to the Greek Islands tomorrow for a whole month.' I could not help wondering if her reaction would have been quite so casual if she had fallen over on the day she returned – with nothing but a bleak English winter staring her in the face.

As we bowled home up our street I remembered how excited I had felt the day before we went to Switzerland many years before. When 'tomorrow' is going to be gorgeous, the things which happen 'today' don't have the same power to hurt. Suddenly I realised it was that very concept which made it possible to be at peace even though life was uncertain. I felt I had seen into Heaven back in 1982; I knew it was going to be wonderful. In comparison, the pain and problems of the present seemed so much less important. If I felt that this life was all we had I would have been outraged by having it spoiled. Instead I have always been conscious that it is only a fragment of our real existence – a prelude to a 'tomorrow' that is going to be even better than the Greek Islands. Later when I described that incident outside the supermarket to Tony, he said it also explained the way he felt.

Chapter 12

Far from making life seem unimportant, the proximity of death seemed to have the effect of making life feel extremely precious. Just believing that 'tomorrow' is going to be good was not enough for Tony and me. We have always thought that 'today' should be fun as well! Looking back over those six years which followed our move to town I can see they were actually very rich and satisfying. We discovered this fulfilment in the most unexpected places. To explain, we must go back to 1985, the year after we left Mayfield.

'May 5th, 1985   Went to Gillingham Hospital in ambulance to be fitted for the ghastly contraption. Apple blossom breathtaking. Had very embarrassing moment on the way home.'

I had been horrified some weeks before when the doctor suggested I might find a wheelchair useful sometimes. I must have looked it, too, because he smiled and said, 'I'll make the arrangements and then you can just get Tony to pop it somewhere for emergencies.'

'I'll get him to "pop" it in the cellar,' I thought grimly, 'and that's where it'll stay.' The thought of people seeing me in a wheelchair appalled me. It felt like the ultimate humiliation.

'You might just as well have one,' said Lyn. 'After all, they are free!' So she had persuaded me into going to Gillingham Hospital, the distribution centre for our district, even though I had no intention of ever using the 'ghastly contraption'.

My morale was instantly boosted by the fact that all the

other passengers in the ambulance had either lost a leg or had no legs at all. Mine might not work too well but at least I still had two of them.

At the other end of the long day, when I was finally taken back to the ambulance, all the other occupants were proudly clutching their new artificial legs. Conversation dragged a bit on the way home. We were all tired out from sitting for hours in a waiting room. When we got stuck in a traffic jam, I made a feeble attempt to lift the atmosphere by saying brightly:

'I hope I get home before my kids arrive back from school. They're always so hungry you'd think they had hollow legs.' I stopped, scarlet and prickling all over with embarrassment as I looked round the ambulance. There was a pregnant pause and then they all burst out laughing and waved their hollow legs at me. After that we swapped hospital horror stories and cracked jokes all the way home. I had been forced to spend most of the previous year either in a hospital cubicle or in bed at home. So this was the first time I had encountered other disabled people since I met Madge at Burrswood. She had said then, 'It's a lot more companionable being with your own kind.' As we joked our way home in that ambulance we certainly seemed to have so many things in common even though our handicaps were different. There was no such thing as 'being one up' on them because I had two legs. We all lived with physical problems and that gave us an equality which instantly created a bond.

About that time the doctor also decided regular physio-therapy would help me. Those sessions at the Kent and Sussex became the focus of the week. The exercises were fun, but it was meeting the other people which did me far more good. As we talked we discovered how many little daily nuisances we shared. Perhaps you can only laugh about things like a leaking catheter and twitching limbs with other people who understand them from personal experience. Other people often say, 'I know how you feel,' but how can they, *really*?

One day I had a phone call. A man with an attractive voice asked if he could call in and see me.

A week later I heard the same voice talking to Lyn downstairs and I expected her to show him through the door. Instead a head suddenly appeared through the bedroom carpet and then a wheelchair emerged from the lift.

The next hour was a sheer delight – John turned out to be one of those fascinating people who cut straight down into the deeper issues which lie below ordinary conversation. He had lost a leg but could no longer have a 'hollow' replacement because of severe arthritis in both his hips. That did not stop him from being a lay reader in his church and spending the rest of his time working for a charity.

Remembering my own struggles with acceptance I asked him if he too had experienced trouble coming to terms with his disabilities.

'After my accident I used to lie in hospital worrying myself silly,' he replied. 'You see my wife had recently left me and I thought, "How am I ever going to bring up two little girls with only one leg – and hold on to my job?" I was a factory manager at the time. The sister knew I was fretting so she would say, "Don't you worry, John, people manage marvellously without legs these days." Then the doctor came round and he said the same thing. When the physios started telling me how wonderful artificial legs were I got a bit browned off – it was easy for all these people to talk – they still had their legs! What did they know about it anyway?

'When Sister told me the chaplain was coming to give me a pep talk I felt that really was the end.

'"I suppose you've come to tell me there's a verse in the Bible which says I ought to like losing a leg," I growled at him when he arrived. He didn't say a word, he just rolled up both his trousers and showed me two tin legs! I listened to everything he said after that. Old man Shakespeare knew what he was on about when he said, "He jests at scars who never knew a wound".'

About the same time as I began the physiotherapy I started to write each month for a magazine called the *Vital Link*. It is specially designed for disabled people who share a

Christian faith, and it has a surprisingly large circulation both in this country and abroad. My pieces were mostly humorous accounts of life from 'where I sat', and I had no idea that through them I would be tapping into a hidden network. Friendship is as vital to disabled people as anyone else, yet so often their handicaps make it difficult for them to get out of their homes to meet people.

The magazine provides a 'meeting place' from which individual friendships begin. Suddenly I found I was in contact with all kinds of different people who have remained my close friends ever since. Some cannot hold a pen so they 'peck' out their messages on a computer keyboard. Others prefer the phone, and many dictate messages to one another on cassettes. I made a bad mistake when I typed my reply to Norma's first 'letter'.

'Please don't ever do that again,' said her next cassette. 'My neighbour had to read your message aloud to me, and he doesn't understand what it's like to be blind.' Neither did I, of course, but although we all had different handicaps there was still that inexplicable bond. One letter said, 'I live in a block of flats in Twickenham and since my arthritis got bad I don't see anyone much. Only my sister-in-law who fetches things in for me. I love writing letters even though my hand has got so bad now.' Another one from a lady called Ellen, in Bristol, said, 'I'm rather glad Christmas is over, I only saw one person all week, my home help who popped in to see if I was all right.' Ellen and I have been in touch frequently for four years now and she always encloses a book of stamps, 'just in case you run short'. I have to confess I often did and Tony hated the sight of our phone bill, but I needed all those people and I felt they needed me.

Until the day when I met all those 'legless' men in the ambulance, I was not sure quite where I fitted in the world any more. Outside my bedroom windows people hurried down the street to work or took their children to school across the park. Yet I felt separated from that world of 'well' people by my circumstances. Once I stopped shying away

124

from contact with other people with handicaps I discovered my new identity group.

The 'ghastly contraption' was the other good thing which came out of that day in Gillingham Hospital (although I would never have believed a wheelchair could possibly be described as a good thing). It did indeed go straight into the cellar that very day, in spite of loud protests from both Lyn and Tony.

'You're being thoroughly pigheaded over this,' he said. 'Don't you realise it would mean you could come shopping with us or out in the park?'

'People might stare at me,' I replied mulishly.

'Well, you could always stare back at them, couldn't you?' put in the ever practical Lyn. They were right as usual. By then I could only get about the house by holding on to the furniture, and going out was virtually impossible because I could only walk a few yards. My precarious balance also made falling over a hazard. My pride kept me a prisoner in my own home until Duncan's school sports day two months later. I wanted to go so badly and see him run.

'The chair's the answer,' said Tony, but I wasn't so sure.

'How would Duncan feel?' He still did not find my handicaps easy to accept and that puzzling barrier was still between us. In the end he agreed to let me appear in the chair; he was tipped to win the flat race and his desire for me to share his glory outweighed his embarrassment. It did the same for mine.

As Tony pushed me towards the group of other parents, I remember feeling very self-conscious. Somehow the wheelchair made my problems much more obvious and cut me off from the 'well world' more decisively than walking sticks had done. People looked as if they were thinking, 'poor thing', and pity was the last thing I wanted. But it was not nearly so bad as I thought it might be. Sitting there felt like being a real mum again and the chair with its head support was very comfortable indeed. The support was necessary because my

125

neck muscles always seemed too weak to hold my head up for more than a few minutes.

Duncan covered himself with glory in every race he entered and just as we were beginning to wonder how soon we could politely slip away, the mother's race was announced. As I watched sprightly mums kick off their high heels, discard their babies and hurry towards the starting line, I suddenly noticed Duncan thundering towards me.

'You're going in for this race too, Mum,' he said firmly, 'I'll push your chair.' I knew instinctively that this mattered to him and whatever the consequences I was going to have to look as if I was loving every minute of it. We have a photograph in our family album which proves that I managed it! We did not win the race, but neither did we come in last – we collided with another mum, knocked her flat and proceeded to pip her at the finishing tape.

After that day I began to see that the wheelchair really could be a liberating experience rather than a final defeat. Although I was never 'confined' to it and seldom used it in the house, it made going out much easier. Family activities such as picnics and Christmas shopping became possible again. So did trips to the seaside, so long as we chose places with a promenade and not a sandy beach. Over the years Duncan must have pushed me for miles through the country lanes. Even at ten he was as strong as a bull elephant and our only problem arose when it rained. The spokes of my umbrella kept poking him in the eye!

There were certain irritations attached to the wheelchair, of course. Other people seemed to have an unfair psychological advantage as they towered above me, and constantly looking up at everyone made me feel strangely devalued. Besides, it gave me a crick in my neck! The worst thing of all was when people only talked to the person pushing me.

There was one place I would never go in the wheelchair and that was church. I hated the thought of being stuck conspicuously in the aisle. Even when it meant Tony practically had to carry me in, I insisted on sitting in the back row so I could use the wall to support my head. Churches can be some of the most difficult places for wheelchairs, with flights of steps, rigid seating and unsuitable loos. In fact, going out anywhere in a wheelchair has its problems, as we discovered the day we went to London.

In the autumn of 1988 I was going through a very good patch of health. So when Tony asked me what I would like to do for my birthday treat, I replied promptly, 'Go to London on a train and look round Harrods.' Tony looked pleased; we had not been able to have a 'jaunt' like that for years.

'I'll take you out to lunch,' he promised. I was secretly a little daunted by that. I hated eating in public, for I often dribbled and dropped food down my front. 'We'll find somewhere nice and quiet,' he said, sensing my embarrassment.

On a frosty October morning we set off for the station with Naomi, who kindly consented to come in case I needed help in the loo. It was at the ticket barrier that we encountered our first obstacle.

'You can't take her in your carriage, you know. She'll have to go in the guard's van.'

'All on her own?' said Tony.

'There aren't seats in the van for passengers on this line.'

Finally Tony decided to put the chair in the guard's van and he and Naomi manhandled me into an ordinary carriage – one pulled me from above while the other pushed hard on my back end. Not a pleasant experience for any of us, but we were determined that nothing should spoil our day.

At Charing Cross we finally managed to hail a taxi but, just as it approached, a small van pulled up to the pavement in front of us. The cockney cab driver wound down his window and shouted in a voice which caused every head in the station forecourt to turn in our direction,

'Can't you see I've got a bleedin' cripple 'ere?' We laughed helplessly all the way to Harrods. We would have preferred to go to the opera, which had always been our treat in the old days. To do anything like that with a wheelchair, however, is not so easy. I could sit in an ordinary seat only if the back was high enough to support my head. Sometimes when we took the children to a cinema or theatre I was told I could not go in with them because I constituted a fire risk! It was possible occasionally to ring in advance so they could remove a seat to make room for me, but the hassle involved seemed to spoil the fun somehow.

Browsing round Harrods more than made up for everything, but by the end of the day we were all so tired we were glad to get back to Tunbridge Wells station. As he extracted me from the train, Tony could have done without the sight of a huge flight of stairs.

'Don't worry,' said Naomi. 'There's a notice over there, saying "Disabled please ask staff".'

We did.

'It's no good asking now,' said the ticket collector as he chewed a grimy matchstick. 'You should have asked in London, shouldn't you?'

'Should we?' said Tony.

'Then we could've diverted the train to the up line.'

'I don't suppose we'll be going to London again,' said Tony wearily, 'but if ever we do, I'll remember that. Isn't there a lift?'

'Oh yes, but it hasn't worked since I've been here.'

'Then how do you suggest I get my wife home?'

'Well, I'll have to find at least four people to help,' he said without offering to do so.

As Tony and Naomi finally humped me ignominiously up those stairs, I wondered why the station bothered to display that notice at all.

It was 1986 when I received the mark II version of my wheelchair and it was the best present anyone ever gave me. That summer my brother Justyn came to visit us from Canada where he was living. One evening he drove me out to Ashdown Forest for a leisurely gossip in the sunset.

'What's the hardest thing about all that's happened to you?' he asked me unexpectedly. Under Lyn's tutorage I had

128

become so used to concentrating on the good things that I was floored for a moment, then I said, 'Never being alone in the open air. When I get stuck over something I'm writing I would love to be able to go out and think it right through.'

'But you have the wheelchair,' he said. 'Couldn't you go out in the park?'

'Wheelchairs aren't that much help when your arms are basically as weak as your legs. If you can't propel yourself more than a few yards you've got to have someone pushing you. It's being *alone* that matters.'

'What you need is a kind of modern Bath chair,' he said thoughtfully. 'I'll buy you one.' He couldn't afford it, but I knew a little thing like that would never stop him.

One of those three-wheeled scooters was what I wanted, but after I had been assessed by the occupational therapists they insisted I needed the head and arm support of a battery-operated wheelchair.

It was a hot summer evening when the 'Bug' finally arrived. Naturally the entire family wanted to show me how to operate it, but I insisted on going into the park alone for the maiden voyage. I could see a face at every window of our house and I certainly gave them plenty of entertainment. The joystick was very sensitive and until I became used to its light touch I shot madly in all directions.

The shadows were lying long across the grass in the park that evening and suddenly I was alone. I remember stopping for ages to watch little green caterpillars swinging down from the oak trees on the end of their silky threads. I could sit and enjoy them for as long as I liked without boring my pusher. The exhilaration of being able to propel myself along effortlessly again was also something I will never forget. So even when I capsized in a drain I insisted on my right to independence.

The Bug gave me back my freedom. I could go and fetch Richard from school every day and take Minty for walks in the park. Once again I could go to the supermarket – but sadly not the post office, because of those unfortunate steps.

The reference library and bank were out of reach for the same irritating reason. All the same, my world became much larger. Not only could I enjoy our own park but across the main road lay Calverley Gardens and a little farther away was Dunorlan Park with its great wide lake. No longer did I have to rely on 'imaginary' trips to beautiful places.

I will never forget the sheer joy of the first autumn after I had the Bug. In the mornings the cobwebs on the park gates were spangled with dew, they looked like diamonds in the sunshine. The following spring I sat so long one day looking at the early crocuses that the kindly park keeper came over to ask if I was feeling all right. Later in the year he was most concerned when he found me crying over a cluster of yellow-brown toadstools growing out of a tree stump.

The arrival of the Bug brought me one disappointment, however. I imagined it would open up a contact with the people I 'knew' so well from my bedroom window. 'Now I can just go up to them and start chatting,' I thought happily. 'They'll relate to *me* now and not only to my pusher.' Sadly I was wrong about that. Many people looked away when they saw me coming towards them. Very few people, except our friends from church were willing to make a relationship of any kind with me. Probably it was only embarrassment, and it is something which disabled people just have to learn not to mind.

Even if the Bug proved to be a barrier with some people, it was a definite bridge to others. Older people for instance always had time to stop and talk. The parks were full of them on warm days and the stories they told of life in two wars were a sheer gift to a writer. So were the men whose only home was the park. Calverley Gardens seemed to be a gathering place for a surprising number of homeless people and I found their unusual angles on life very refreshing. They were always highly amused at the sight of Richard riding home from school on my lap, steering the Bug for me. Few things have ever touched me more than when they pooled their meagre resources to buy him a Christmas present.

One day I received a letter with a Maidstone postmark. It was from someone I had never met, but she told me she had read an article of mine in *Family* magazine.

'I've decided to give a little coffee morning,' she said, 'and I wondered if you would be well enough to come and give a talk.' She was a churchgoer, she explained, but many of her friends were not. 'I think they would enjoy it if you told us why you still believe in a God of love even though you are now disabled. There'll only be about fifteen of us and the babies can just crawl round our feet.'

My first reaction was, 'Oh no! I don't want a lot of bright, well, young mums looking at me as if I was some kind of a circus freak. What have I got in common with them now anyway? Perhaps I had developed a kind of 'them and us' mentality towards what I called the 'well world'. Then I read her letter through again and noticed one small sentence at the very end. 'One or two of them are having a bit of a rough time at present.' I remembered that coffee morning back in Mayfield. Behind the masks some of them had been hurt by life quite as much as I had. It had shown me that people are not only disabled by losing their health – losing a partner, a job or a home can be crippling too. So I wrote back and said I would go.

After that I used to say yes to speaking engagements like that whenever I was in a good patch. So often I seemed to meet people who felt their lives were toppling like a house of cards. I had felt like that once, and the very last thing I would have wanted then was to hear people talking about faith who had never suffered much in their own lives. (Like the clergyman who told me to think positively when all the pain he had ever known was a headache.) In my wheelchair I did not constitute a threat to them. The same bond of understanding which exists between physically handicapped people also exists between any human being who has suffered loss. The very greatest satisfaction of all for me was seeing other people find that same personal friendship with God that I had discovered was such a delight.

Travelling was always terribly tiring, so perhaps my greatest contact with people like that came through letters.

The first book I wrote for Hodder and Stoughton described the struggle we had to hold on to our faith in God during the first two years I was ill. After it came out in 1986, I was amazed by the flood of letters it produced. 'I knew *just* what you were talking about, I felt the same after we lost our daughter of eight . . .'

'I read your book a few months ago when my marriage was breaking up. I seemed to go through so many of the same experiences as you did . . .'

People simply wanted to 'talk' to someone else whose life had buckled too, and many of the letters grew into friendships which I still value today. Letter writing has always been a great hobby of mine, although in the pre-computer days it was my crazy spelling mistakes which gave my recipients the most pleasure! Soon I found I was writing more than a hundred letters a week and through them I 'met' some quite remarkable people.

Life during those years after I fell in the muddy bog was definitely satisfying: watching the children grow up, seeing Tony enjoying life, the interest of our church, writing, speaking engagements and the letters. Before we left Mayfield Tony had seen the need to leave our dream world behind and begin to build something new. The pleasure we had once taken in the beauties of the countryside had been replaced by relationships with people.

PART
THREE

Chapter 13

'January 1st, 1990   New Year, new decade. I wonder what it will bring.' (Had I known I would have been extremely surprised!) 'Thank you Lord that they [the family] all love you in their own ways and that they are all happy and doing well.'

That Christmas, as we had all sat around the table together, I smiled as I remembered how often I had worried that my illness might ruin their lives and destroy their faith. My fears had proved to be ill founded.

Tony's career was most successful and his name in the world of education was known and respected nationally. Sarah had gone to Oxford and taken a first in history despite all her problems with school when I was first ill. She was now happily married to Paul and still at Oxford doing her PhD. Justyn, at twenty-one, was still full of laughter and love of sport, and it was hardly surprising that he was doing a degree in physical education. Jane was happy and very settled in a job at the town hall. She had her own bedsit up the road but frequently came in to see us. Naomi at seventeen was working hard for her A-levels at the local grammar school and Duncan, although he was only fifteen, looked down at us all from his six foot four inches. He was already playing rugby for his county and fitting golf and weight training into his spare time. Richard was twelve and enjoying life at Tony's old school in Tonbridge. What more could a wife and mother possibly want? Those prayers with Father Keith at Burrswood back in 1982 had certainly been answered.

Yes, life was being good for them all, but for me, the year which proved to be the happiest ever actually started rather badly. That winter the Peace-joy kept being yanked away like a warm blanket on a chilly morning. In September I had been very ill again but there were several other things which disturbed me.

The first was writer's block. The previous Easter I had begun to write a novel, my first for the adult market. That was something I had always wanted to do and it had been such fun at first.

The idea for the book had come when I looked out of my window about five one morning and watched our milk lady plodding up the terrace under the amber street lights. As she left her trail of gleaming white bottles on the Victorian doorsteps I had thought how cosy all the houses looked. It was not long since the Lockerbie air disaster when the fuselage of a bombed aeroplane had hurtled from the sky and wiped out most of a street in a little Scottish town. It suddenly occurred to me that something like that could just as easily have happened here, in Tunbridge Wells. All at once I began to imagine myself standing out there in the park watching the destruction of my own street.

Two hours later when Tony finally woke, he discovered me sitting up in bed beside him tapping furiously at my keyboard. I was so completely involved in the scene I was describing he had a job to convince me the street was still intact outside our bedroom windows.

'This is going to be the last chapter,' I told him. 'I'll start the book a year before the crash, then I can watch the people in the terrace while the sand in their hour-glass trickles away.'

'For goodness' sake don't base the characters on our real neighbours,' he pleaded, 'or they'll sue us!'

'Do you remember old Mrs Pennington? That tiny sparrow of a lady who died one morning when I was in the Kent and Sussex? Surely it would be quite safe to make her the main character. I always thought she'd make a good heroine. She

136

can live in this house, too, so long as I make it much grander than it is.'

'Here we go again,' sighed Tony, but he was smiling as he went off to make some tea.

After years of writing non-fiction, I found the following four months such fun. Those imaginary characters actually became more real to me than the flesh and blood people in the world around me.

Then came the illness in September 1989. It was not a serious flare-up. The doctor had allowed me to stay at home, even though that meant a lot more bother for him. District nurses came in during the day and night to look after me and the catheter, and administer the morphine sulphate plus all the other drugs. By Christmas I was still struggling my way up out of it again, and I did not seem to be making much progress. The sheer effort of getting better had sapped all my creativity and the novel had completely died on me. The characters still lived in my head, but I did not seem to have the energy to transfer them on to paper. I could not even face the thought of the letters which I usually enjoyed so much. Ever since I had started writing seriously, six years before, I had always worked from the time the children went to school in the morning until they returned at teatime. That winter was different. I seemed to spend all my time staring aimlessly at my keyboard.

During the time I was in bed in the autumn, for no apparent reason I had started to think about healing again. It seemed strange to me that I had been in contact with so many ill and disabled people over the last few years and yet never once had I seen any of them miraculously healed. Many of the books I had once read so avidly implied that it often happened. At first it was not my own healing I was thinking about, but I did so much want to see some of my friends getting better. So one day I wrote this prayer in my diary.

'October 1989   Lord I've seen people begin to get better after prayer gradually, but never seen anyone healed miraculously like in the New Testament. Please let me see someone I know healed suddenly like that.'

Not long afterwards I was introduced to a tall, graceful young woman called Julie Sheldon. Someone told me she had been a ballerina. As I looked up at her from my wheelchair, I realised she was the answer to that prayer. She had been seriously disabled by a neurological disease called Dystonia, and had become so ill she had actually been dying in a London hospital. Just a few months before we met, someone had prayed for her and now she was completely well again.

'So it does still happen,' I thought with a strange mixture of emotions. We were talking away as if we had known each other all our lives, but inside I began to think, 'If it could happen to her, then why didn't it happen to me? What did she do to deserve this?' She looked so poised and well standing up there above me with her husband Tom smiling happily in the background. I felt so envious that it took several days before I managed to regain my equilibrium.

'Don't you dare start getting all wound up about healing again,' said Tony firmly. 'It's not worth the hassle.'

'He's right,' I told myself and pushed the thought of Julie Sheldon away.

Then came a very nasty blow – the loss of Lyn in January. Government cut-backs meant she was no longer allowed to give the time she felt some of her clients badly needed. We were all right when her hours were reduced because friends from church took on the ironing and other vital jobs, but she worried about elderly and lonely people who were not so lucky. The strain of watching their distress was too much for someone as conscientious as Lyn. Tension led to back trouble and she was finally forced to leave social services altogether. The whole family missed her unspeakably – even though the home help office sent along someone else. After six years no one could replace Lyn and her sense of humour.

She found a job in a shop at the end of our road and insisted on coming in every lunch-time to sort out my pills.

She refused to hand over to anyone else that intricate responsibility.

The next disturbing thing happened in February. When Sir Harry Secombe's TV programme, *Highway*, visited Burrswood he wanted to interview several people who had received miraculous healings there. He also wanted to talk to someone who patently had not been healed. So I was invited to take part in the programme.

As Grace drove me over to Burrswood I was scared at the thought of cameras but wildly excited at the prospect of meeting Sir Harry. As a little girl I had never missed listening to him on the *Goon Show*. As I grew up I watched all his films and collected his records. Would meeting such a famous star face to face actually be a disappointment? I wondered, as I was pushed into Dorothy Kerin's sitting room. It was swarming with TV men that day, fussing over lights and cameras, but the moment Sir Harry walked in there was silence. His personality filled the room yet he managed to make everyone there feel important. Our interview took only a few minutes and then he sat chatting to me as if we had been friends all our lives. Two days later he sent me such a huge bunch of flowers I felt like a film star myself.

Eagerly I waited to see the recorded programme, but the experience did not turn out to be enjoyable at all.

It was screened on Sunday, February 4th and only Duncan was at home to watch it with me. The others had all gone out after they had set the video and exhausted the jokes about Mum being a telly personality. Things had been very strained between Duncan and me for some time. I had always thought it was his love of physical fitness and speed which still made my limitations such a trial to him. Somehow we always seemed to rub each other up the wrong way and I had been praying that God would heal our relationship.

As we sat together watching the familiar buildings and beautiful grounds of Burrswood, he suddenly said vehemently, 'I hate that place. I'm never *ever* going back there.' I looked up at him sharply and suddenly I remembered a furious little boy of six, kicking and screaming at me because I could not come home with him and make his world safe again. A flood of bad memories came surging back into my mind as I remembered his being dragged away down the corridor. Before I was ill he had been a happy, carefree little boy, but he had changed into someone who was tense, fearful and very often angry. 'Perhaps I was wrong at Christmas,' I thought. 'One of them really did suffer permanent damage through all this.' Duncan has always shared Tony's reserve and I do not think we had ever spoken to each other about that terrible visit to Burrswood.

'You must have thought I let you down so badly,' I said. He remembered it all vividly as we began to talk that evening. Why, I wondered, had we never done this before? I should not have allowed him to bury all those memories for so long. We were still talking when everyone else came home to watch the video.

That evening an invisible wall which had separated us for so long seemed to crumble away. Later, Duncan was able to tell me something which helped explain why it had been there in the first place. When I had been in hospital that first time in 1982, someone who was looking after the children told him that my illness must all have been caused by his bad behaviour. I was so horrified I thought at first he must have made a mistake, but when I told Sarah about it she remembered the incident well. She never thought Duncan would believe a remark which had been made under pressure by an otherwise kindly adult who was trusted and loved by us all. No wonder he had been so disturbed! Those few words had helped to devastate his childhood and caused the two of us years of anguish. When he saw me at Burrswood he must have felt personally responsible for my problems and it could have been guilt which had made him appear so angry with me ever since.

Talking to each other that night in February paved the way for an entirely new relationship to form between us and he has been a totally different person ever since. Healed relation-

140

ships are far more important than healed bodies – and I will always believe that.

In spite of the good which came out of watching that television programme, the incident, like the others that winter, left me strangely vulnerable and unsettled.

While all these things were attacking my peace of mind, something very strange was happening. People, many of whom I did not even know personally, began to feel the urge to pray specifically for my recovery. One particular church in Eastbourne, St Michael and All Angels, which I had never visited, prayed for me each Thursday at their healing service. Other churches did the same. I did not ask for this and in most cases I did not even know they were doing it. I kept the promise I had made in the back cover of my Bible never to ask for healing again. Yet I subsequently discovered that separately and spontaneously other people began to pray for me at that time.

The writer's block was still just as bad by March.

'I'm totally stuck,' I told Tony gloomily. He had taken me out in the Bug for one of our rare trips to a local café, but even that did not seem to be cheering me up.

'Give up then,' he suggested, 'and start on a new book.'

'But this is something I want to do so much,' I told him, In fact I felt I would never be a real writer until I had done a novel.

'The trouble is I just can't decide whom to kill!' I burst out loudly. All round us respectable Tunbridge Wells faces looked round in startled horror.

'Just a book I'm trying to write,' I murmured foolishly to the woman at the next table. Tony threw back his head and roared with laughter, but it was not funny really. During that year I had become so fond of some of my characters that I could not face putting them through such a violent death! Particularly not Rosie, who was really Mrs Pennington. The plane was never intended to destroy the whole street so I found myself wanting it to land on the irritating people while it narrowly missed the nice ones. Of course it never happens

141

like that in real disasters. The good suffer just the same as their nasty neighbours. So if this novel was going to be true to life I was going to have to be ruthless.

'I think you should go away for a few days' break and think the whole thing through,' said Tony decisively. 'I'll give that nice little place in Alfriston a ring — it's off season so they won't mind giving you all the help you need.'

On March 11th he deposited me and my word processor in a tiny little room containing just a chest of drawers and a bed. But the view from the window was all that mattered to me. The village of Alfriston is tucked into the folds of the South Downs a few miles from Beachy Head.

'I'm not coming back until you've sorted yourself out,' said Tony, who always sounds gruff when he minds about something. We hate saying goodbye.

The following morning I was sitting propped up in bed drinking a cup of tea when quite suddenly into my mind came the words, 'I want to heal you.' As usual there was no voice, but the impression was just as vivid as if I had heard one. After the surprise had worn off, I decided I must have imagined it. I felt rather annoyed as I picked up my diary and scrawled, 'March 12th Alfriston. Came here to write end of novel. Completely blocked ... Lord *help me*, all I can think of is healing ... Don't let me waste time and money here ... I must work on Claire today.'

After another cup of tea I pulled the keyboard towards me and forced myself to think about 'Claire' and her imaginary hairdresser's shop. But I could not get those words out of my mind.

'This is ridiculous,' I thought. 'I've got to stop this silly wishful thinking.' I did not want to let myself get upset yet again, as I had done after I met Julie Sheldon. If healing was not going to happen for me, then I ought to concentrate on the things I could do and not hanker after the rest. At night I had often dreamed I was walking in the bluebell woods again, but I tried hard not to let thoughts like that enter my mind in the day. My peace was too important.

Somehow I did not seem to be able to banish the thought so easily this time. All through the morning I struggled with it, while the book made no progress at all.

'I'm not going to get all unsettled again,' I thought furiously as I remembered the months of rising hope and bitter disappointments which had led to the muddy bog.

By midday, in spite of my resolve, I was beginning to think, 'Suppose it wasn't imagination, after all? What if it really was God's voice I heard? How would it feel to be better again?' All the thoughts I had held down for so long began to bubble up ecstatically as if someone had pulled the cork from a champagne bottle. 'Stop it!' I told myself firmly. 'Or you'll never survive the disappointment.'

All that day I wrestled with myself and my faith. How could I know if that inner voice was really God speaking to me, or simply my own subconscious telling me what I wanted to hear? The whole idea was ridiculous anyway. The DSS did not ever bother to have me assessed regularly any more. The last doctor who examined me had signed me off indefinitely. They obviously did not expect me to get better. But all the evening those words, 'I want to heal you,' kept on disturbing me. I had been so sure God wanted to use me as a disabled person, so why should he suddenly change his mind?

'Please,' I whispered just before I finally put off the light. 'Don't mess about like this. If it *is* you talking, how can I know for sure? Please give me a sign.'

When I woke early the following morning I knew without doubt what the sign would be. And hastily I wrote it down.

'March 13th   I must wait patiently for someone to come out of the blue who will confirm this, pray and lay hands on me and I will be well. Thank you Lord, I want that . . . I thought you could best use me . . . from a wheelchair. I give you permission to use my life *anyway* you want. It's yours.'

After I had finished writing that entry, I still was not sure what I was supposed to do now. I knew without a shadow of doubt that I was going to get better, but how would I meet this person? Should I go somewhere like Lourdes, or Burrswood? Ought I to try and get in touch with them by going to all those healing services again? Then once again I felt he was telling me clearly what to do. In large letters I wrote four more words right across the page: 'I must wait quietly.' Obviously he was going to do the rest. At last I lay back on my pillows again with a sigh of relief. It all seemed so simple now.

'But it's going to be hard to wait quietly,' I thought. 'I won't even be able to tell Tony.' I knew silence was vital all the same. When this mysterious person arrived, I needed to know they had been prompted by God. If I went round telling everyone, how could I be sure it was not me who had planted the idea.

It might seem easy – just being asked to sit and wait for a divine messenger, but I honestly think it would have been far easier if I had been sent on a long and difficult pilgrimage – with dried peas in the tyres of my wheelchair! Waiting is so hard for someone as impatient as I am. Fortunately for my sanity, as I was sitting looking out of the window later that day I suddenly found myself thinking about the book again. I knew exactly how the story should end. Almost without thinking I pulled the keyboard towards me and started typing. After that the whole book came alive. On Friday afternoon, when Naomi came to fetch me, I was working at it in a positive frenzy.

She had always been such a good friend to me. When Lyn was not there I relied on her for all the little personal things. It had often worried me that she might find it difficult to leave home with a free mind.

As we drove back towards Tunbridge Wells I wanted to say, 'Now you'll be able to go to university in October without worrying about me.' I bit back the words, however, and chattered about the weather.

Chapter 14

The next few weeks seemed like a race against the clock as I lay in my reclining chair typing away madly. I tried hard not to think about healing too much because I felt under an obligation to finish the novel and hated the thought of my characters being still-born before I could kill them off myself!

By May 4th my friend Liz had altered all my bizarre spellings and the manuscript had been retyped and sent off to the publishers. I felt bereft all that day, I always do when I finish a book. It feels like handing a new-born baby over to strangers and not even being sure if they will be kind to it. By five o'clock the following morning – May 5th – I was wide awake and feeling more like celebrating. Tony had woken up early too. He put my Bug in the back of the car and we drove out to his allotment. He enjoyed digging away up there before the world woke up and I loved going with him because it was right where the edge of the town met the country.

As I rolled along the lane at the side of the allotments, with Minty sitting on my lap, I realised the book had absorbed me so completely I had not been out like this for weeks. The little rows of houses soon disappeared behind us and fields took their place. It was a perfect morning, the sun was still only hedge high, a pale pastel ball in a hazy yellow sky. When the lane began to wind through a wood the new green beech leaves formed a tunnel for us. Through the fence on either side I could see carpets of bluebells stretching away in all directions. Suddenly I remembered a day in Fir Toll Wood, eight years before, and I stopped with a jerk. Bluebells were symbolic for me. When I had been up here last winter, this little wood had been all drab browns and greys. Now it was transformed. My life too was going to be changed out of all recognition by the same creative force.

My heart began to beat quite painfully with excitement. Minty, bored by the inactivity, jumped down and trotted off into the woods in search of rabbits. 'I'll be able to go with her soon – and smell the bluebells too,' I thought and then realised something else. 'If I'm well there'll be no more reason to stay living in town. We won't have to make do with just an allotment. We could find a little house by a wood like this, wake up to hear the birds singing the dawn chorus every morning.' As I sat there with the tears streaming down my face I remembered an ancient Jewish poem from The Song of Solomon I had learnt as a child:

> Rise up my love . . .
> and come away.
> For, lo, the winter is past,
> the rain is over and gone;
> The flowers appear on the earth;
> the time of the singing of birds is come.

When at last Tony came looking for me, I had a difficult job convincing him I was actually crying with happiness.

The weeks which followed were filled with an indescribable feeling of expectation. I began to devour the four gospels as if I had never read them before in my life. The person of Jesus seemed to step out of the pages as I read about the different ways he had helped people. 'This is the one who said he would heal me,' I kept on thinking. Although I knew he was going to send 'a messenger' who would lay hands on me, Father Keith had made it quite clear all those years before that it was not human hands which heal but the power of God flowing through them. The arrival of the messenger was obviously very important to me, however, and every time the phone or doorbell rang I jumped. Was this the 'person' come at last? Often I used to lie in bed and picture to myself how it would all happen.

'When I'm prayed for,' I told myself, 'I mustn't be surprised if nothing happens at first. It will only be the start of a long slow healing process that's sure to take at least two years.' I never even considered that healing might be instant.

One day in the middle of May when Tony took me out in the car to see the Kentish apple blossom I nearly gave everything away. Without thinking I said happily,

'Oh, won't it be lovely when I can drive myself!'

'Don't start that again,' he said firmly. 'You know you've been told you never will.' The effort of keeping silent was becoming increasingly hard. I longed to share it all with him but hesitated, not only because of those words, 'wait quietly', but also I felt he was too close to me emotionally. The strain of knowing my whole way of life could change at any minute grew greater by the day. It was a strange blend of apprehension mixed with wild excitement. Like waiting for the birth of a first baby which has been longed for over many years.

As May went by I became oddly emotional and kept on bursting into tears for no obvious reason. Something seemed to have removed the lid which had held down all the darker things of the previous eight years. At inconvenient moments I would suddenly remember hurtling through the hospital corridors in that wheelchair, Tony's face on the far side of those cot bars and days when the pain filled every part of my body.

One evening in May I had to speak at the local branch of the Mothers' Union on the subject of 'The Disabled Mother'. All went well at first as I sat in my wheelchair at the front of a large church hall. I was talking about home helps and invalidity benefits when suddenly I thought of Duncan screaming at Burrswood. What had it *really* been like for my family to have a disabled mother? I paused and swallowed hard. Rows of kindly faces smiled encouragement, but I wanted to shout, 'It's been hell sometimes!' Fortunately I did no such thing, but to my unutterable embarrassment, tears began to ooze down my cheeks. They were all very nice to me, but as someone drove me home I vowed I would never speak at another meeting again in my life!

That night I wrote a note in my diary, 'May 24th   When the Lord has yanked away your Peace-joy, you can't face being disabled any more.' For years I had felt that inner contentment was a gift which had made all the difficulties possible. Now it had been taken from me, I simply could not cope. Yet I had the distinct feeling that it had to be removed before the healing could take place.

It was rapidly becoming clear to me that I could no longer go through this experience on my own. I needed detached and professional help and I felt God understood that and would not mind if I confided fully in my friend Diana Priest. She is a health visitor, a trained Christian counsellor and also totally discreet. She believed my strange story and every week she came and allowed me to talk through all my feelings, hopes and misgivings. She felt the 'patches of darkness' which kept on enveloping me were a cleansing experience and as we prayed about them it seemed as if I was being healed on the inside first. Together we also faced the practical changes that healing would make. Illness had felt like a prison at first, but during long sentences even prisons can begin to feel like safe places. I often remembered that TV programme we had once watched about the old prisoner who had looked forward to her release for so long, then as the time drew near had begun to wonder how she would manage to survive back in the outside world. I did just the same. Illness has its perks too, and Diana helped me plan coping strategies for life without them.

As May went by and the bluebells were nothing but limp leaves and white stalks I was beginning to be a little anxious. We were thinking about summer holidays by then and wondering if the farmhouse we were renting in Scotland would be suitable for me. I so hoped I would be well before we went away so that ramps, wide doorways and downstairs bedrooms would not need to concern us this year. Tony and

Duncan were talking endlessly about the golf they were planning. Once I had played for Essex off a single figure handicap and I wanted to beat them both hollow this summer and not spend it sitting in car parks.

'May 30th   Lord Jesus I swing from great hope to helpless despair . . . When are you going to heal me?'

Things went badly wrong when my patience began to wear thin and the old achievement-orientated person inside me asserted herself. Surely it can't be right, I reasoned, just to sit back and 'wait quietly' for a gift to be given to me. I must have got that bit wrong. One day I watched a video of the film, *Brother Sun Sister Moon*. I was very moved by the sight of Saint Francis of Assisi struggling to rebuild a ruined church – barefoot in the snow. My body felt to me like a tumbledown ruin too. Perhaps I was supposed to work at its repair with the same kind of tenacity as Francis had displayed. Surely God helps those who help themselves. By that time I seemed to be over the effects of the last flare-up and was beginning to feel better physically. So I began to force myself to walk about as much as I could with my two sticks. My 'bagy sagy' muscles, as I described them in my diary, worried me greatly. So when a friend of mine with MS happened to show me a simple little exercise routine, I decided to try it. It had been specially worked out for her, but it pushed me right up to my pain barrier and then beyond. Tony watched my efforts with a sigh of resignation. He had seen me pushing myself like this before and he knew what the end would be. He was maddeningly right as usual. By the beginning of June I had lost ground again badly and was exhausted, painridden and discouraged.

'June 9th   Went to Burrswood . . . Made myself go up to communion rail with only my sticks. *So* tired had to go straight to bed.' That was the day I finally realised the healing was not something I could achieve myself. I was also feeling so ill again by then it was hard to keep on believing I would ever be healed at all.

A certain date on the calendar was approaching at a terrifying speed. 'June 13th All-day conference on suffering, Haslemere.' The thought of it terrified me. How was I ever going to cope with a two-hour car journey, let alone having to talk in the morning *and* the afternoon. What if I broke down as I had at the Mothers' Union meeting? And what could I possibly say about suffering? All I knew about it was how much it hurts.

So I decided to ring Viv Jackson who was organising the day in Haslemere.

'Look, I'm very worried about Wednesday,' I began. 'I seem to have lost my nerve somehow.'

Viv was sympathetic but she was in a difficult position. 'I've asked some very special people to come,' she pointed out. 'Some of them are physically disabled but others are hurting in all kinds of ways. Please try and come if you possibly can.'

'But I don't feel I've got anything to say,' I pleaded. 'I'm not a vicar who can produce a sermon on demand.'

'They'd hate a sermon,' said Viv. 'Just come and tell us how you found your own faith.'

On June 11th when the dreaded date was only two days away I decided to put the morning aside to prepare what I was going to say. Conventional prayer seemed quite impossible that morning, so I tried a method I learned when I was eight: My school friend Mary had been dying of cancer. I wanted to pray for her so badly, just like I wanted to pray now, but the right words entirely escaped me. That week a visitor was staying in our home, an elderly clergyman called Harding Wood. He was so small his round blue eyes seemed to be level with mine. He was the kind of person children trust instinctively so I felt I could tell him all about Mary and my inability to pray for her. The fact that his pockets were always full of butterscotch made him a particularly comforting father confessor.

'Does your mind make pictures when you shut your eyes?' he asked me unexpectedly as we both sat there sucking happily. I told him it did – all the time. 'Well then, let yourself

150

see God sitting up on a great big throne, like a king in the clouds. Can you see him?' I nodded vigorously. 'Now look at yourself walking towards him leading Mary by the hand. That's all prayer is, just taking her to God so he can smile down on her. You don't need words so it's easy, isn't it?' I wasn't sure until I had another butterscotch, then I said,

'But I thought it was Jesus who made people well.' Uncle Harding's blue eyes twinkled as he bent towards me and whispered, 'I'll tell you a secret. Jesus is actually part of God – dressed up in a man's outfit.'

Since I had been thinking so much about Jesus and healing, I had often pictured him as I prayed over the last few weeks. I never saw Him clearly, just a fuzzy outline in a background of beautiful countryside. That morning as I thought about all those people in Haslemere I tried to picture Him again, but no image would come. He did not seem to be there and all I could see was myself standing in an expanse of empty space holding out a little wooden begging bowl. It was cracked and dried out by the sun and when I finally gave up and opened my eyes I felt just as empty as the bowl.

Later that day the phone rang. It was a friend who has a great interest in the subject of healing. Some time before, I had heard she was spending regular days praying and fasting for my recovery. In fact I had wondered for weeks if she could be 'the person' I was expecting. So when she asked if she could come over and see me about something important, hope began to surge like water in a canal lock when the sluice gate is lifted. 'This is it! At long last,' I thought as my gloom was blissfully transformed.

By the time she arrived I was positively stiff all over with anticipation. She talked about many things but she never once mentioned healing. 'Perhaps she's shy,' I thought, and decided to give her a little prompt.

'If ever you felt you had some kind of a message for me, you would tell me wouldn't you?' I said, as I tried to keep my voice casual.

'Of course I would,' she replied kindly. 'I'd tell you straightaway.'

She went at last and I lay back in my chair and allowed myself to cry. Actually I felt like howling so loudly the whole street would hear. For the first time I really began to doubt that experience I had at Alfriston. The entry in my diary that night is obviously a desperate attempt to think positively.

'June 11th ... when she had gone felt so let down and sad but suddenly realised I would face far more temptations if I am healed. While I am ill I am a nobody to most people. Get healed and I could begin to think I was a somebody. Proudly think I had done something to earn my healing. I'd lose you then. "God ... give me yourself for you are enough for me" (Mother Julian of Norwich c. 1400).' Then later, (probably during the night) I added this telling little postscript at the bottom of the page. 'I cannot face *not* being healed. The thought is terrible.'

Chapter 15

It was pointless lying there trying to sleep. Even when I did manage to doze off it was only to dream I was sitting dumbly in front of all those strange faces in Haslemere. I might as well leave Tony to sleep undisturbed by my restlessness and go downstairs. It was only about four o'clock when my lift glided down in the eerie grey of the dawn and even the sparrows in the park had not begun to chirrup. I sat in the corner of our lounge huddled in an old car rug. Inspiration simply must come soon, or I really was going to sit in that church completely dumb, like I had in my dream. Perhaps one of 'Uncle Harding's' picture prayers might help me?

What happened next subsequently changed the way I look at most things in life, yet I still do not quite understand it. It could have been a daydream, a particularly vivid figment of my imagination – or it might have been something much more special. For once I did not feel I was 'making' the pictures myself; they happened independently all around me in vivid colour and quite remarkable detail. I was standing before a great high throne and once again I was holding up a pathetic little begging bowl. Behind me I was conscious of many other people, row upon row of them. Somehow I knew they were the women I had to address that day in Haslemere. I looked round curiously and my reaction was one of horror. They looked emaciated – their faces twisted with suffering and etched by stress. They too, were all holding out empty bowls in a silent appeal. They reminded me of an Oxfam poster and I thought, 'people in prosperous English towns don't look like that'. Then I remembered the real expressions hidden behind those masks at the coffee morning in Mayfield. Were these people also coping with secret griefs and private anxieties? How could I possibly pray for them when I knew nothing about their circumstances?

So I turned back to that great throne again, 'Please . . .' I began, but the words just petered out. It was then that I noticed someone else was kneeling beside me praying for those people in a way I never could have done. He seemed to know each of them intimately and slowly I realised it was Christ Himself. I could not see His face because His head was bowed but as He prayed in detail for each one, I knew He was crying. He obviously cared so deeply for their suffering.

For a very long time I just watched. Then, as I looked into those haggard faces once again, I realised I still had nothing to say that day and nothing to give. My own bowl was just as empty as theirs.

Then, to my great relief I noticed that Christ had stood up and was moving along the rows of people. He stopped beside every one and gently cupped His hands round those suffering faces. At last I saw His face. It was beautiful, quite beyond description. Even if I could paint like Michelangelo I would never be able to convey that look of tender understanding. Somehow His smile reminded me of all the different people who helped me during the years I was ill. Father Keith, George Swannell, Tony, Lyn, and so many more. Into each empty bowl He put something different. I could not see what it was but I knew it represented the answer to the personal and private need of each of them. Yet some people, when they saw Him approaching, threw their bowls down on the ground and turned away. I longed for Him to come and fill my bowl but before He reached me the scene gradually began to fade away.

For a long time I sat there motionless. There was nothing I needed to do that day – or say for that matter. It was all going to be done by someone else.

154

With a sudden surge of relief I shot towards my lift and pressed the up button vigorously.

'Don't worry any more, Tony,' I said as I poked him. 'Everything's going to be all right today in Haslemere. Something wonderful's going to happen.' The only thing worrying Tony at that moment was being woken out of a deep sleep!

Getting me ready to go out anywhere always seemed to involve the entire family and we did not have long that morning to go through the routine. Penny (the wife of our minister in Mayfield), was coming for me at half-past seven. Tony checked the wheelchair, and fixed the head rest while Naomi found my surgical collar. I rummaged in my bag to make sure I had the necessary nappies, spare underclothes and gloves to keep my icy hands warm. Even Lyn turned up to see I took the usual arsenal of pills with me.

'Here's your dark glasses, Mum,' said Duncan as Penny's car drove into the road, and Richard handed me my walking sticks.

'You don't really look fit to go,' said Tony as he looked anxiously at the colour of my face. 'It's going to be a bad pain day isn't it?' He was right. Now I had a cast-iron excuse to ring Viv and cry off entirely, but nothing was going to make me miss whatever was going to happen in Haslemere that day.

Penny was not alone. In the back of her car I could see Jo and her guitar. She has a wonderful voice and had agreed to sing some of her own compositions to lighten the proceedings that day. I could hardly wait to tell them both about what I had seen that morning.

'Everything's going to be all right today,' I said as we left the town traffic behind us. But the two-hour journey seemed terribly long, and as the pain increased my optimism waned.

'You know, Penny,' I said, 'I've been so silly recently. Three months ago today, I actually thought I was going to be healed. I even wrote in my diary that I should expect someone to come to me soon – right out of nowhere – and tell me so!'

155

'Never mind,' said Penny soothingly. 'It's just getting through today that counts.'

When they had finally heaved me and all my paraphernalia through the doors of the church, I liked the feel of the place. People were milling about in all directions, serving coffee, setting up a bookstall, showing people to their seats and checking microphones. Yet there was a stillness about the place in spite of all the activity. Viv gave me an anxious look and hastily I explained what I had 'seen' early that morning.

'Don't worry,' I whispered. 'It's not up to me today.' But my confidence wavered a little when the programme began. As Jo was singing I sat beside her in my wheelchair and looked out across the rows of people. 'I've been very stupid,' I thought. The faces looking back at me were not gaunt and miserable, they were all beautifully made up and capped by immaculate hair styles. I felt ill suddenly, with that clammy, cold, breathless feeling that comes just before you faint. Terrified I would start being sick, I tried to breathe deeply and concentrate on Jo's singing.

But I did not faint, and as I began to speak I actually forgot about the pain in my head. I did not do my talk well, the words and ideas came out muddled — just as they always did on a bad-pain day, but it was as though it was not me they were hearing at all. Mascara began to run as the masks melted away. I knew Christ was touching people and satisfying their needs just as surely as I had seen Him doing so earlier that morning.

When the clock on the wall told me it was time to break for lunch, I said, 'Are there any comments or questions just before we close?'

Right in the very front row sat a young woman who must have been in her twenties.

'Excuse me,' she said quietly, 'but what is actually wrong with you? Ever since I wrote that resolve in the back cover of my Bible. I had never liked talking about details like that. So I simply said, 'Oh I've had five attacks of encephalitis',

156

and tried to hurry on to someone else. But she went on talking and I noticed that she looked acutely embarrassed.

'I've never had anything like this happen to me before,' she mumbled, 'I've only been coming to church for a few months, you see. But I feel God is telling me to tell you that you are going to get well.'

It had happened. I do not know how I knew, but there was never any doubt in my mind that here was the person I had waited to meet for so long. I caught Penny's startled expression right across the room and Jo stirred in her seat beside me.

'Would you mind saying that again?' I asked. 'You see I've waited three months to hear someone tell me that.'

As she nervously repeated herself, I burst into tears of sheer relief. Jo stood up hastily and played another song while people all over the church looked as if they were wondering whatever was happening.

'She has to pray and lay hands on me,' I thought. 'It was all part of the promise.' But as everyone began to surge in the direction of the refreshments I lost sight of the young woman completely. A buffet lunch was served in the basement. Obviously there was no way I was going to get down there, but food was the last thing I cared about just then. So many people wanted to be prayed for that Viv, Penny, Jo and I were all kept busy. Then as the hands of the clock crept towards half past one I began to think, 'Suppose that girl doesn't come back for the afternoon session?'

But she was there. Right in the front row once again. During the afternoon I told them some of the things I had discovered recently as I re-read the gospels. It was so easy to talk about Jesus – I felt I had seen Him only that morning. While Jo was singing a final song, I kept looking at the young woman in the front row. For three months I had been wondering what kind of person would be sent to me. I had envisaged someone like Father Keith or George Swannell. 'She looks so young,' I thought. 'I'll have to move very quickly at the end of this song, or I'll lose her again.' I do not remember feeling excited, I merely felt compelled to reach her before it was too late. When Viv had finally closed the meeting, I pushed the back wheels of my chair violently in the direction of the front row, with a complete disregard for intervening toes.

'Please,' I said breathlessly, 'would you mind praying for me?' She gazed at me in silent dismay, so I continued, 'I'm sure if you laid hands on me, I would be healed.'

'Didn't I make it clear,' she said looking down helplessly at me, 'all this kind of thing is new to me? I've only been a Christian for just over a year. I don't have a gift of healing. I wouldn't be able to pray for you properly.'

'Please . . .' I said urgently, but just at that moment someone came up to offer me a cup of tea. By the time I looked back the young woman was gone and I just caught sight of her disappearing out of the back door of the church. My emotions seemed to have been shooting up and down like a yo-yo for the last few days, but at that moment they reached their lowest point. Never have I wanted a cup of tea less in my life.

'She's gone!' I said.

'You mean Wendy?' said the lady with the tray of cups. 'She's probably gone home to feed her baby.'

But Wendy had not gone home. Instead she had dashed in search of one of the church leaders.

'You'll have to come and pray for this woman,' she said as she burst into his office. 'I'm just not the right kind of person to do it.'

'I'm sorry, but I can't pray for her either,' he said when he had managed to help her explain. 'You have been given this conviction, so you must pray.' With that he sent her back into the church to find me.

Many people had gone home by then, but quite a crowd still lingered and they formed a circle around us.

'What do I do now?' asked Wendy diffidently. I seem to remember someone telling her to place her hands on my head and they added, 'Just allow God to use your hands as you pray, then his power can flow through them.'

She was so nervous I could feel her hands shaking and I really cannot remember the words she used except that her prayer did not contain any flowery theological phrases. She simply asked Jesus Christ to make me well.

I felt absolutely nothing. No sensations nor even any emotion. Just the matter of fact satisfaction of knowing a job had been done at long last.

When I opened my eyes no one gazed at me to see if I would stand up, because no one really expected that I would (– except Wendy.)

'Well,' I said when people began to drift away, 'I'm not going out of here in a wheelchair.' The moment I moved I knew something was different. Whenever I had been sitting upright for a time my muscles used to stiffen until they locked me rigidly into that position. Before I could attempt to stand, it used to take a very long time and a great deal of effort to get my knees and hips to straighten themselves out. That day I simply stood up.

Privacy was the first thing I felt I needed. I wanted to feel myself all over and discover exactly what had happened to me. So I walked away from everyone and hid in the ladies' loo. It was probably the first time anyone had ever locked themselves in there in order to waggle their limbs about, jog on the spot and discover just how hard they could grip the toilet roll!

When I finally emerged, Wendy had disappeared, and I hadn't even had the chance to say goodbye. It was three months before I met her again and learnt the reasons why she was so reluctant to pray for me. Her story fascinated me so much I have written it in an appendix at the back of this book.

Chapter 16

People often ask me what I felt like on the journey home from Haslemere. I felt nothing. Just numb. The healing had come, I knew that, but I had been wrong when I thought it would be the beginning of a long gradual recovery. Frankly I was a little afraid and my mind could not allow itself to register the full implications of what had happened. It focused on all kinds of trivial little things instead.

Penny and Jo seemed to understand that I did not want to talk about it and I think we giggled rather a lot and discussed Mayfield gossip. Towards the end of the journey I began to wonder what I would do when I arrived home. The decision, however, was not hard to make because the following day Naomi was going to be eighteen. Personal birthday cakes used to be a tradition in our family, but the collection of iced aeroplanes, castles and crinoline ladies were all on the far side of the eight years and we had made do with frozen gateaux from the supermarket for a long time. Why shouldn't I make her a real home-made cake? That was what I wanted to do more than anything else.

In my mind's eye I could see it already: pale pink butter-ice enclosing fluffy sponge cake. I'd go straight in and make a start the moment I got back. For some crazy reason the cake seemed to matter more than the feelings and reactions of the family. The words 'wait quietly', still seemed to bind me and I thought it would be better to let people see the change in me for themselves. How much better it would have been if only I had talked to them at once.

Tony and Naomi were ready to 'deal' with me as soon as Penny's car turned into our road. The routine was always the same: after going out all day I hardly knew where I was with pain and fatigue so they would push me up the ramp at the side of the house, bundle me into the lift and help me straight to bed. After more pain-killers and a warm drink they would depart to let me sleep off the exhaustion. That sometimes took twenty-four hours.

I will never forget their faces as they stood at the front door watching me pull my wheelchair up the front steps towards them.

If I was making this story up I would describe how I floated euphorically round the house all the evening smiling angelically. It was not like that at all and everyone keeps on reminding me just how bad tempered I actually was. I am not sure if all the excitement had been too much for my equilibrium or whether I was simply trying to re-establish my independence and mark out a new territory.

Whatever the cause, I marched straight into the kitchen and proceeded to shout at the boys for leaving their school bags and blazers in a heap on the floor. I had not possessed strong enough chest muscles to shout for so long the effect was enormous!

Gom, who had been like a mum to me since I was a baby, was cooking the supper. She had looked after the house all day, yet for some reason I felt the need to blast her for doing the chicken in the wrong way. She was so overjoyed to see me looking so well that she forgave me, but she must have gone home feeling rather crushed.

Naomi is a very gentle person, and my outburst made her so indignant she retired to her bedroom refusing to come down again all the evening. Tony also disappeared in the direction of his allotment. He always goes there when I'm bad tempered.

Far from feeling repentant I was actually glad I had managed to clear the kitchen for action. Only Duncan had the pluck to stay near enough to watch my antics. Sadly the cake was not the success I had envisaged. Obviously I was badly out of practice and it refused to rise, so I had to substitute a swiss roll I found in the fridge. Then when I tried to disguise it with plenty of icing I put in too much cochineal and the resulting shade was positively revolting! I remember pulling the shelf out of the oven and squealing with pain. It was a hard way to discover I could feel things again.

'No one's going to eat a cake that colour,' said Duncan as he licked out the bowl.

'Never mind,' I snapped. 'Help me blow up some balloons.'

'Help? I'll have to do them all,' he grumbled, 'because you know you can't blow.'

'Just watch me,' I replied. When I climbed on to the dining-room table to tie them to the light above he stood gazing at me like someone who has woken from a dream to find it was real after all.

It was while I was setting the birthday breakfast table with an elaborate flower arrangement and all the best silver and glass that Tony came home with an armful of lettuces. He gave me an odd look and then dashed out again to a church meeting. Undeterred, I decided to celebrate one of the greatest days of my life by doing two large baskets of ironing.

Early the following morning I groped towards the chest by my bed for the plastic container of pills Lyn had left for me. By five in the morning pain-killers were always necessary. Sleepily I scooped them out of the pot and lifted the glass of water. Then I stopped. What was I doing this for? I wasn't in pain and my muscles were not stiff at all.

Beyond the curtains the sun was already shining but it would be at least two hours before Naomi wanted her birthday breakfast. I could go out and have the whole world to myself if I was careful not to wake Tony.

It seems ridiculous to say the thing which gave me the most pleasure on that first day was putting on my tights. Shoes, however, were more of a problem. I had only needed one pair and naturally they never wore out. As I put them on I discovered that my feet seemed to have changed shape and made the shoes feel distinctly uncomfortable. 'I'll have to borrow a pair,' I thought, and went downstairs to find some. At the bottom I stopped and looked back up the staircase – then I ran up and down it several times just to make sure I really could do it.

Outside our kitchen a set of shelves had become the dumping ground for everything which 'might just come in handy one day'. I rummaged about among the jumble and at last pulled out an old pair of walking shoes that had once belonged to Tony's Auntie Enid. They did not fit too well, but they were better than nothing. 'I'll sort all this mess out later today,' I promised myself happily and, grasping my two sticks, I went towards the front door. On the step I paused. Why did I need my sticks? I wasn't dizzy and my legs no longer felt like wobbly jelly. But the sticks had been part of me for years now. 'Two legs are better than four' was another family joke. I couldn't possibly go out without them, it was bad enough facing the world without the wheelchair.

Leaving those sticks behind was surprisingly hard. It was the first of a series of psychological barriers I had to go through. The moment I began to walk down the street without them I felt a tremendous surge of joy. I couldn't remember walking right along our road alone since the day I set out for the post office almost exactly six years before. The contrast was so great I did a kind of dancing hop all the way down the pavement. Then suddenly I stopped, overcome with shyness. It was only just after five, but a man was walking towards me and I felt oddly undressed without my props. My embarrassment grew even greater when I realised I knew him well. He had been a good friend over the years – the fact that he could not talk and I could not walk very well never seemed to hamper our relationship. Now I wanted to bolt up a nearby alley and hide, but it was too late; he had recognised me and was gazing at me quite mystified.

'I went to a church near Guildford yesterday,' I said breathlessly and without preamble, 'and now look at me, I came

163

home completely well.' (Why I felt I could tell him and not my own family I simply cannot imagine.)

His confusion slowly gave way to an enormous smile and his whole face went bright red. I could see he wanted to say so much in response; instead he began to leap up and down on the pavement with sheer joy and the noises he managed to make were some of the most moving sounds I have ever heard.

Somehow I felt too embarrassed to go into our own park. Even at that early hour too many people might look out through their lace curtains. So I hurried across the road to Calverley Gardens because I knew the roses were just coming into bloom. Looking at the flowers in that lovely park had been one of the joys of my life, but smelling them again was glorious.

No one was about, so I began to run across the smooth sloping lawns making crazy footpath patterns in the dew. Minty ran along behind me looking distinctly cross. She was getting old now and enjoyed riding on my lap in the Bug. Her patience snapped when I climbed on to a low wall just to see if I could balance. She yapped indignantly as I ran along the top and jumped down again just for the thrill of feeling my body move through the air.

Then the early morning joggers began to arrive so I felt it was time to be a little more discreet. Leaving the gardens I hurried across town in the direction of my other favourite place, Dunorlan Park. Walking along the familiar pavements felt so strange, because I could see so much more than I had from the Bug. Gardens that had always been hidden behind hedges were suddenly accessible. As I was standing on some-one's wall to enjoy their display of delphiniums a passing milkman gave me a very odd look.

The park gates were locked when we arrived, but Minty drew my attention to a gap in the fence and we were through it at once! Dunorlan is a beautiful place. Often on bad pain days I had tried to distract myself by an imaginary walk round the huge lake and under the fine old trees. 'This time it's for real,' I thought in sudden awe.

As I jogged round the lake I thought about all the times I had ridden sedately along the same path in my Bug on a Sunday afternoon. During my recent attempt to 'get myself better' I had even tottered painfully a little way on my sticks. This present freedom felt intoxicating.

Early morning mist like a duvet covered the surface of the water and made the ducks and geese appear positively ethereal as they glided about. Suddenly I stopped still in the path. The sun shone warm on my face and the scent of the newly-cut grass wafted over me. I was quite overcome by the extent of the gift God had given me. All these little things I might have taken for granted if I had never lost them at all.

'Thank you,' I whispered. 'Thank you so very much.' As I stood there I had the distinct impression that the face I had 'seen' looking so sad and full of compassion the previous morning was smiling now. Sharing the pleasure with me. The words of an old hymn came into my mind and I began to sing them softly.

> Were the whole realm of nature mine,
> That were an offering far too small,
> Love so amazing, so divine,
> Demands my soul, my life, my all.

Yes, I thought, even if I could collect up all the most beautiful things I have ever seen to give to Him, still they would not be adequate.

Feeling totally overwhelmed I began walking round and round the lake. After the fifth circuit I realised my feet were covered in blisters. Not a very remarkable thing considering the ancient shoes and the distance I had covered. What mattered to me, after years of having 'dead' feet, was that I could *feel* they were sore!

Panic greeted me when I arrived home.

'Wherever were you?' the family demanded furiously.

People receiving the severe disability allowance at the highest possible rate simply do not disappear for long solitary walks. They had been about to ring the police.

Breakfast was a silent meal. Only six of us sat round the table that morning. Jane and Sarah had their own homes by then, but Justyn had arrived home from college a few days before. None of us quite knew what to say.

It was not until after they had all dispersed that I found the envelope. I had completely forgotten that, just as we were leaving Haslemere the day before, the woman who had been sitting next to Wendy had given it to me with a message scrawled in the corner. I had been too dazed to do more than stick it in my bag but I pulled it out now and looked at it more carefully. It simply said, 'Revelation 22.10.' Feeling rather puzzled I looked up the obscure passage in the last book of the Bible. 'Do not keep the prophetic words ... a secret, because the time is near when all this will happen.' How she could have known that I needed to hear those words I shall never know, but I took them to mean I could now tell everyone what had happened to me.

No one was left in the house by then, except Justyn. He was splashing about in the bath, so I rang the home help office. Never have I felt quite such a fool in my life.

'We ... er won't be needing any more help from now on,' I began diffidently. The clerk obviously thought I was my own mother-in-law because she said sympathetically,

'Oh, I am so very sorry. When did Mrs Larcombe ... er?'

'Oh I'm still here,' I said hastily, 'this is me talking. I'm just better, that's all.' I was pretty sure she would be ringing my doctor as soon as I put the phone down to discover if I was now mentally ill on top of everything else. 'He's someone else I'll have to tell,' I thought, but how could a woman who was healthy enough to go early morning jogging ring the surgery and ask for an appointment? The necessity was removed when he actually rang me himself later that day.

'I see you are due for a smear test,' he said. 'When can I come round and do it?'

'Oh you mustn't bother,' I said nervously. 'I'll come to you.' There was a pause and then he replied, 'Oh I see, you'll get Tony to bring you on a Saturday morning.'

'Oh no, I don't want to trouble you then,' I answered. 'I'll just make an ordinary appointment next week.'

'Well I'll tell my receptionist to look out for your chair so they can help you in,' he said kindly, and I was smiling as I put down the phone.

Naomi was in the middle of her A-levels but that day she was free so Justyn drove us over to Sevenoaks for a birthday lunch with Tony's mother. On the way I told them everything. Their reactions were typical. Naomi was quiet and thoughtful – she always is. Justyn was jubilant.

'I'll work out an exercise programme for you, Mum,' he said, 'to get your muscle tone back.' After I had taken him on a very long, fast route-march through the deer park at Knole that afternoon (in spite of the blisters) he recognised his programme was not going to be necessary.

Once Duncan realised I was completely well he looked as if some great burden had finally been lifted from him. His excitement was enormous. A few days later I remember him sitting in the kitchen rocking on the back legs of his chair.

'Mum,' he said, 'if God can do this for you, he can do anything.' We have never had the slightest difficulty in getting him to church ever since!

Richard's initial reaction was more restrained. It was almost as if he was shy of me at first because I had changed so much. When I raced him home down the street a little while later he said:

'I've never seen you running before, Mum.' He had, of course, but he was too young to remember. 'It feels like living with someone else,' he added wistfully.

Jane came round for Naomi's birthday tea that afternoon, and she looked as relieved as Duncan when she saw me. I often wonder if the same unfortunate remark was also made to her. It would explain many of the problems she went through after I was first ill.

Sarah was due to come and stay with us a few days later. She needed to spend three weeks in a particular library doing some research and our home was more convenient during that time. I did not ring to tell her beforehand but took her out to lunch as soon as she arrived off the train from Oxford. She was thrilled. The coffee and sandwiches we had in the café felt more like champagne and caviar.

After I told Tony on the evening of Naomi's birthday, his reaction puzzled me greatly. For just over a week it felt as if we had gone back to those dreadful six months when he withdrew from me. I was so upset and frustrated I felt like hitting him! Part of it was shock. He had not had the three months of mental adjustment I had been given. Some of it was fear. He had lived through too many disappointments before, when my condition had improved a little and then relapsed again. Of course I had never been well like this since before 1982. He could see I was drastically different but still he was afraid to let himself believe that for a while. So during that first week he was maddeningly silent, but I ought to have expected that really: he never has allowed his most important thoughts and feelings to show.

It was very unusual for us all to be together at once like we were for those first three weeks (Jane came in frequently). It was vital that we had that time. We needed a chance to unpack this wonderful gift we had been given as a family.

Duncan had been right about the birthday cake – no one risked it except the park sparrows who must be colour blind! However, by Saturday my confidence in the kitchen was beginning to return.

Naomi had not planned any special celebration for her eighteenth birthday – parties had been out of the question for the last eight years. Instead she was asking a few of her school friends round on Saturday evening for a pizza from the take-away.

'Let me do a real dinner party for them instead,' I suggested. She looked annoyed.

'You'll only get tired half-way through and I'll have to do it all,' she said woodenly.

But it turned out to be a blazing success. It took all day to prepare a four-course dinner for twelve but what a pleasure to cook without all the old clumsiness and frustration.

It was while I was in the middle of all the preparations that Lyn came in to see me.

'What are you doing?' she demanded, looking round the cluttered kitchen. 'You'll go and drop something.'

As I told her what had happened at Haslemere I wondered what pithy utterance she would produce to add to the family archives. For once she was speechless and had to sit down at the table for some time. At last she gave me a fierce hug and said:

'I hope you'll still remember to take your pills.' I confessed that I kept on forgetting them – there was no pain to remind me. In fact I never took any of them again in spite of Lyn's protests. Many of them were the kind which should have caused withdrawal symptoms, but I never suffered from any kind of trouble at all.

In church on Sunday I discovered I could sing properly again and I stood and bellowed out the alto part until I was hoarse. All our friends were thrilled for us once they realised what had happened, and a few weeks later the Minister put on a special service of celebration.

By Monday I had stopped feeling embarrassed about my new body, and that was just as well. Every time I stepped out of the house during those first few weeks people would bang on their front windows and wave as I walked by. The lady at the baker's shop left a queue of customers and ran out into the street to congratulate me, and a complete stranger stopped me in the supermarket and said, 'Excuse me, have you a sister in a wheelchair?' People who had once looked the other way when they saw me, smiled and said 'good morning'. Others I had never met sent me bunches of flowers.

On Tuesday I went to collect my child benefit allowance.

It is difficult to describe how I felt as I ran lightly up the steps of the post office and stood effortlessly in the lengthy queue.

Chapter 17

It seems strange that the rest of the world was positively delighted by the change in me, yet at home we were having some problems of adjustment.

In spite of the obvious pleasure and relief, some of the family were also angry at first.

'Why weren't we told back in March too?'

'If God can do this now, why didn't He make you better when we were smaller and needed you more?'

One evening about a week after Haslemere I went for a long walk round the lake in Dunorlan Park with Sarah.

'What *is* the matter with them all?' I demanded. She has always been the spokesperson for the family.

'We can't cope with the change in you. It's just too much,' she replied. 'Everything about you is different – even the colour of your skin. We've forgotten how to relate to a mum who doesn't need our help, who wants to be in charge of the kitchen and bosses everyone around.'

In my enthusiasm to do everything again myself I had been far from tactful. Since Lyn had left the previous January, the children had been in charge of cleaning the four bedrooms on the third floor of the house. My lift did not go up that high, so the mess I could not see had never bothered me. When I did see it, however, I was horrified by the mouldy apple cores, dead coffee mugs, dust and dirty washing. One morning, when they were all safely out at school I went up with the vacuum, scrubbing brush, disinfectant and quantities of rubbish bags. They were horrified when they came home.

'We'll never find anything now, Mum,' they said reproachfully.

The whole household was in chaos during that first week. Naturally over the years various routines and arrangements had been developed to keep everything running smoothly. Now suddenly every one of those structures was upset, roles were changed, responsibilities altered and identities lost. Soon no one, including the dog, seemed to know what they were expected to do and when!

Probably I was just as prickly as they were. I resented it bitterly when they would keep trying to help me out of chairs, in and out of the car or up steps. It was only force of habit after so long, but telling them I did not need their help made them feel confused and redundant. Sometimes people can become so used to caring for another person that when the need is no longer there they feel bereft.

There was something else happening to us all at that time which I could only explain when I remembered the experience of some friends of ours. The father of the family was killed tragically in a motorway accident. The three children supported their mother wonderfully until two years later, when she married a doctor. The children all liked and trusted their step-father and loved their new home. Just when everything should have been happy again, all three of them seemed to go to pieces emotionally. They had managed to live through the time of prolonged strain without showing any signs of distress. It was not until the problems were over that they could face up to the painful memories. During that first week or two I think all seven of my family went through a very difficult patch emotionally. Richard put it into words when he said:

'I keep remembering horrid things which make me sad.'

Sarah was able to tell me one evening how angry she had felt when I first came home from hospital in 1982. It explained the awful rows we had during the last two years in Mayfield. She, like everyone else, had thought I was going to die. When she heard I was coming home after all, she was delighted – until I arrived.

'You weren't Mum any more, you crawled round like a cross old woman, saying "fetch that", "do this", "move the other". I wanted to be all carefree and "teenagerish" but instead I had to be everyone's mother – and yours. I used to think it would have been so much easier if you had died, and then I felt so guilty.'

If I had my time over again (and I am profoundly glad that I won't), I would never underestimate the destructive power of buried guilt.

While we were all readjusting to each other indoors, life outside the home continued to be marvellous.

'Wednesday June 20th Incredible day, had to speak at Christ Church, Southborough. They had billed me as a mum in a wheelchair. I hope they weren't too disappointed when I walked in and stood up to speak at the front of the hall for a whole hour! Told them all what happened only a week ago today at Haslemere. I've lost eight pounds since then with all the running about.'

A friend of mine called Jane was there at the meeting that day. She had been coming to do my hair regularly for some time, so the sight of me startled her not a little. A year before she had been cutting my hair one day when I noticed her face reflected in the mirror. She looked so sad. Caught off guard she told me how she had wanted a baby for years, but that day her hopes had been disappointed yet again.

When she finished the hair do we sat on my bed and asked God that she would become pregnant. As we prayed I imagined her walking round holding a baby in her arms. It had always been a very deep sorrow to me that I would never be able to hold a child again myself.

She came up to me after the meeting and handed me Hannah who had been born just a few weeks before. I knew she had arrived but this was the first time I had seen her. As I stood there holding that tiny bundle in my arms we both cried with sheer joy.

As far as I can remember it was the following day that I went to coffee with a friend and met a physiotherapist who was staying with her. She was most interested in my story but perhaps slightly sceptical. She wanted to feel the muscles of my arms and legs and, after she had done so, she sat back on the sofa rather hastily.

'This makes me frightened,' she said. 'I would have to work on you for six months to achieve muscle tone like this.'

Friday June 22nd was also an incredible day. My blisters were better so I set off to the shopping precinct to buy a new pair of shoes. I had never allowed myself to think how much I hated shopping in a wheelchair. That afternoon without one was such a contrast. When I walked into the shoe shop, no one stared at me, looked embarrassed or seemed annoyed at the amount of floor space my wheels were taking up. No one smiled patronisingly or bent over me in exaggerated and self-conscious concern. I was just an ordinary customer at whom no one looked and thought, 'Poor thing, but how brave.'

'Can I help you?' asked the assistant and she was talking to *me* and not my pusher. My eyes were on the same level as hers and suddenly I felt like a person again.

The window of the next door shop was full of soft toys, and I went in to buy a present for baby Hannah. While I stood waiting to be served I reached out and touched one of the teddy bears in the window display. The soft texture of its fur was lovely after so many years with hands which felt they were wearing thick leather gloves.

Without really thinking what I was doing I touched the velvet ears of the teddy's rabbity neighbour. Then explored the long silky hair of a toy dog. I threw all caution to the wind after that and began running both hands at once over every different fabric I could reach – just for the fun of it. A reproachful cough at my elbow reminded me how stupid I must look. As the assistant pointed politely to a notice which said, 'please do not touch', I knew there was no way I could explain my bizarre behaviour. So I hurriedly left the shop without daring to buy anything after all.

On the far side of the road was a window full of colourful bathing costumes. Having a bath had been a big undertaking for a long time, sometimes even requiring the help of the district nurse. Gliding effortlessly through deep water had been something I often dreamed about. In I dashed without a second thought and bought the cheapest suit they had on offer. Then I actually jumped on a bus. Fortunately it was travelling in the direction of the swimming-pool but the fun of riding on it was so great that I really would not have minded where it was going.

When I eventually slipped into the pool, it was full of earnest-looking 'keep fit' enthusiasts, swimming up and down in straight rows like robots. They looked slightly irritated by someone who turned wild somersaults, bounced up and down like a dolphin and positively wallowed about in sheer delight. As I looked at the serious faces bobbing rhythmically with the breast stroke, I wondered if they really appreciated the joy of bodies which move through the water totally free of any pain and stiffness. Did they ever think about the people who cannot experience that pleasure? I wanted to shout, 'Don't take it all for granted, you don't know how lucky you are!' I was crying when I pulled myself out of the water. Those first weeks were a strange mixture of ecstasy and grief.

On Sunday June 24th, Richard had to sing with his school choir in a church in Southborough on the outskirts of Tunbridge Wells.

'Let's go for a walk in the country while we wait for him,' I suggested. Tony had been very busy at work during the ten days since I came home from Haslemere, so this was the first time he really had a chance to see me walking out of doors. A path led us through some fields and I raced Minty down the hill, then did my version of a Girl Guides' vault over the stile at the bottom. Perhaps I really wanted to shock Tony out of the daze he had been in for ten days. I forced the pace relentlessly, as we crossed another field and went through the woods so fast I never noticed the trees at all. It was while we were climbing another very steep hill that he stopped. When I looked back at him I noticed that a light had suddenly come on behind his eyes.

'We really do have a future together, don't we?' he said huskily.

That moment was not just one of my 'flashes' of happiness. We both felt it was more like an explosion! We talked solidly for the rest of the afternoon as we strolled at a kinder pace through the buttercups.

'I'll give up my job,' he said. 'We'll sell the house and find a little old farmhouse somewhere in the country.'

'Marvellous!' I replied. 'But how will we live?'

'We'll do bed and breakfast,' he answered promptly, 'and in the off season you'll write novels and I'll write educational textbooks. We'll walk miles every day and have lots of dogs.'

'And a goat,' I added firmly.

When Richard slid into the back of the car he gave us both a searching look.

'Why are you two laughing like that?' he said.

'Perhaps we only just remembered how to,' said Tony. From that very evening the whole family seemed to take their cue from him and all the doubts, fears and negative reactions were dispersed by what I can only describe as a blast of joy.

It is rather exciting to fall in love again at forty-seven, and it certainly makes it less embarrassing if you happen to be married already! It was not that we had ever fallen out of love, but many factors had forced our relationship to become emotionally distant.

Suddenly the whole world seemed to contain only the two of us and I remember wandering round Tunbridge Wells the following Saturday in a daze, hand in hand, while Tony bought me all kinds of new clothes. Neither of us ever wanted to see again the 'sensible' full skirts that are suitable for wheelchairs or the drab easy-to-wash blouses and cardigans.

So we chose colours, shades and styles I had never dared try before and somehow they reflected our mood. As I was hidden in the changing room I could hear him telling the assistant all about how I had been healed, just as enthusiastically as I might have done myself.

One evening Tony had to go up to London to a meeting, and I went too so we could have the time to talk. So many subjects had been taboo when our future was so uncertain. Now we had a great deal of ground to cover and there never quite seemed enough time at home.

We felt as lightheaded as if we were on our first date as we ran hand in hand through the puddles in Regent Street. As we dodged pedestrians and pelted across roads it was strange to realise the last time we had been together in London was the day when the taxi driver called me a 'bleedin' cripple!'

One day the doorbell rang. As I opened it I was confronted by the biggest bunch of flowers I have ever seen in my life. They were from Sir Harry Secombe. 'I cannot tell you how absolutely delighted I was to hear that you are marauding all over Tunbridge Wells on your two feet . . .' said his letter, which arrived the following day. The children pinned it up on the kitchen wall and they show it proudly to everyone.

'You're never in these days, when I come round to see you,' said a friend rather acidly one day. She was right, and her remark made me realise that it was probably just as hard for our friends to accept the change in me as it had been for the family. Others used to say, 'Do be careful', 'Don't overdo things or you'll soon be back in the wheelchair', 'Take a long slow convalescence, go to bed every afternoon.'

'Why?' I thought. 'I'm perfectly well, so I ought to be allowed to enjoy life to the full.' The sheer size of our family had made it necessary for us to rely on a large group of friends for practical help as well as company. We could not have survived without them, yet some wanted to go on treating me like an invalid wrapped up in cotton wool. I knew it was vital for me to escape from that cosy protection. To upset these wonderful people who had meant so much to us was the last thing I wanted to do, but sometimes, in order to recover successfully, it is necessary to override the need of some carers to go on caring.

Looking back now I think I probably behaved rather like an adolescent in my fight for independence and for a while I wanted to shy away from everyone and everything which reminded me of the illness. For instance, I felt I should purge the house of its 'invalid' atmosphere. Every time I opened my desk drawer, the disability pension books were there looking at me. The cupboard was full of bottles of pills. The lift seemed to take up so much room in both lounge and bedroom and I kept tripping over the redundant Bug parked in the corner of the dining room. The day after Haslemere I had put the manual wheelchair in the lift and stacked all my other disabled equipment in on top of it. Large packets of incontinence pads and sheets, spare catheters, surgical collar, walking sticks and feeding utensils. Only the Bug and commode were too big to fit in as well.

'I want to get rid of the lot,' I said about three weeks after I was better.

'You mustn't do that!' said friends in horror. 'Suppose you're ill again.'

'I'm not going to suppose anything of the kind,' I replied, 'and that's why it's all got to go.'

I was goaded into action at last by a fierce argument I had with my three sons one evening when we went to a concert in Tonbridge. We were late, seats were limited and the car park was full. Justyn drove us round and round in a hopeless attempt to find a space.

'Get your orange badge out, Mum,' they urged, 'then we can park right at the front door.'

'But I'm not disabled,' I pointed out.

'You couldn't be prosecuted until you're signed off.' Fortunately a car pulled away just as I was deciding to sit on the badge to prevent them from getting it.

As we sat in the concert I decided that I must take action at once. So I wrote to my friend Jenny in Canterbury, whose MS was making life a little restricted, and asked if she would like the Bug. Then I piled a shopping trolley high with the rest and pushed it all up the hill to the surgery.

I left the more embarrassing things in the district nurse's office with a note asking her to send someone to collect the commode, ripple bed and NHS wheelchair and then waited my turn for the doctor. I had been overcome with shyness the first time I had been to see him less than a week after Haslemere and had not managed to tell him the whole story of what had happened. By the time I paid him this second visit he had obviously heard some rumours about me because he looked up and smiled as if we were sharing a secret joke. On his table I placed my disability allowance books, the orange badge and a vast array of pill pots. (He does not like us to flush down the loo drugs which could be used in third world countries.) He picked up the allowance books and smiled again.

'This has never happened to me before in my professional life,' he said.

'I need to burn the bridges behind me,' I explained. After he had given me a thorough examination he said:

'I just have to thank God with you for what has happened, but professionally I cannot let you send back these state allowances yet, or sanction the removal of the lift. I need to see you completely well for at least three months and I also want to watch the effect of an infection.' I did not feel discouraged because I trusted him, so I made an appointment to see him again in September and went on my way with the empty shopping trolley.

A few days later I began a sore throat. And I was scared. Until my sneezes made the cold obvious I did not even dare to tell Tony. It was like the beginning of a recurring nightmare; we both knew so well what it might mean. Suppose I had only been healed from the effects of previous bouts of inflammation but the virus was still active? During the last

179

eight years, colds and flu had always triggered encephalitis once again. That cold, however, progressed with delightful normality, going down to my chest and making my sinuses and ears painful too. Then it faded away and left me just as fit as I had been before.

Chapter 18

'June 27th, 1990   Wish I could describe what is happening and how life feels now. Like being born anew or putting the clocks back to my twenties and having my whole life over again.'

If ever I should feel miserable in the future I am sure I will only have to read the entries in my diary for the summer of 1990 to disperse the gloom. They are full of all the happy little ordinary things I had not been able to do for so long.

June 30th   Dressmaking all day with Naomi. Made a skirt listening to happy music – Dvorak. So loud blew stereo speakers! Duncan not pleased.'

'July 1st   Went to concert in Trinity Arts Centre with Richard. Sat in an ordinary seat!'

'July 2nd   Minty is having a nervous breakdown! After spending her life sitting quietly by my chair, she is disorientated now I leap all over the house. This morning when I was doing my aerobics she jumped up and nipped me!'

'July 20th   Nearly got killed on road today. Cars used to stop and wave me over in the Bug; keep forgetting I can't just step out like that now. People don't make allowances in the "real world!"'

'July 23rd   Went up the town with Duncan and bought myself some new climbing boots and a rucksack for the holiday.'

'July 24th   Train to London *alone*! Went to publishers (my first publishers, now HarperCollins), had lunch with Christine in a Greek restaurant, talked about publication date for Children's Bible. Got lost on underground, kept going up and down on escalators just for fun!'

'July 25th   Took Richard and Duncan to museum. *So lovely* to go out with them again and do "parenty" things like that! Went on the pitch and putt and we had two rounds.'

The entries which describe our holiday are positively ecstatic, and those weeks in August more than made up for all the previous difficult years. I cannot find a single reference to bad temper.

'August 13th   Two months to the day since Haslemere and what a way to celebrate! Walked twenty-two miles along coastal path. High cliffs, blue sea – and the views!'

The day before, I remember Richard and Duncan watching nervously as I pored over the Ordnance Survey map planning that walk.

'We're not coming with you,' they said firmly, 'you walk too far and too fast for us.' Minty felt the same. She hated the sight of my new walking boots and lay on her back with her legs in the air every time she saw me put them on.

My brother and his family came over from Canada to share the Scottish farmhouse with us. He had imagined a holiday strolling along beside the Bug he had so kindly given me. Instead, I challenged him to a daily round of golf, usually before breakfast. It was marvellous to swing a golf club again and feel that crisp snap as it sends the ball off up the fairway. I did not exactly play to scratch but I did manage to beat Tony and my brother on most occasions – not to mention Duncan and Justyn. My brother stood on the eighteenth green one morning with his hands on his hips and said with a sigh, 'There ought to be a special handicap for people who've had miracles.'

It was slightly ironic that I had to climb my first mountain entirely alone, while Tony nursed a painful ankle at the bottom. It was not much more than a good-sized hill really, but when I stood on the summit and looked at the view across the Solway, I was as happy as if it had been Everest.

On August 6th it was our wedding anniversary and it was

obviously a very special day. Tony took me out to lunch and we sat on a terrace in the bright sunshine looking out over a harbour. I wanted to tell him what his love had meant through all those years but how could I possibly find the words? Humanly speaking, the children's security and happiness is due to him and I am quite sure I would not have bothered to come out of intensive care quite so many times if he had not been waiting for me. Had he left me I would not have been surprised. Madge was right, many marriages do fail because the pressures of disablement are so great. Not only did he continue to cope with me and the family physically, but he supported us all in every other way as well. 'Thanks for doing all those spelling corrections,' was all I managed to say in the end!

We felt we were at a crossroads that day as we sat in the sun. We had been given a new life and after all those years of uncertainty we wanted to spend it together. Quite what we should do was still not clear.

'September 11th Went to the doctor to be signed off at last. As he examined me he kept on saying, "Marvellous!" He says I can drive again when the licensing people at Swansea agree.'

'October 3rd Drove solo.' To attempt a two-hundred-mile round trip on my first day out was probably rather stupid. As a mother, however, how could I miss the chance of taking Naomi to Southampton University to settle her safely in her new room? After eight years, motorway conditions had changed considerably and as I drove along the M25 for the first time I was so scared I was stopped by the police – for going too slowly! Tunbridge Wells in the rush hour was a shock too, and as I sat stuck in a traffic jam, I suddenly realised how much more quickly I could have reached home in my Bug.

'October 16th Lift went. So lovely to see it go!' That morning there had been a ring at the door and Gom, who was spending the day with me, found a small, gloomy looking man on the step wearing a black tie.

'I've come to remove the lift,' he murmured in the tones of an undertaker. As Gom made him a cup of tea he added, 'When did . . . the decease occur?'

'Eh?' said Gom, startled. The little man looked startled himself when I walked in from the park. He explained that his job was a difficult one because he was usually sent to remove lifts only after their user had died. 'I've never had to do it this way on before!' he said, and he actually smiled.

'September 27th Wonderful day. Met Wendy again. She came to lunch with Viv and Penny and together we tried to remember all the events of June 13th. Wendy told us her own story – quite amazing. How I would love to write it sometime.'

Life during this last year has obviously been wonderful, but we have found some things surprisingly painful. For instance, change, even when it is for the better, is still a stressful experience. It is difficult to describe just how great that change really was. Had my recovery been gradual it would not have been so traumatic for all concerned. Suddenly every single department of my life was altered; the way I related to people and how they felt about me; how I spent my days; the way I sorted my finances (we lost more than £100 a week in benefits). The way I looked, felt and moved about. Many of the 'benefits' of illness were suddenly gone too. I no longer had a good excuse if I did not want to do something. People did not make allowances for me all the time, or treat me with unnatural kindness. I had to make my own way in the world and not rely on others to do things for me. It was all so different that sometimes I simply did not know who I was any more or how to handle perfectly ordinary situations.

If it had not been for Diana, my counsellor, I would have been completely at sea. Many helpful books have been written about adjusting to difficult situations; we both felt we were moving into uncharted waters as we faced the problems of adjusting to pleasant ones. One day I remember saying to her, 'I feel as odd as if I was a successful businessman in the

184

City who becomes a woman overnight and has to stay at home all day looking after a horde of small children.'

While coping with a change as large as that, it did not help to find ourselves the object of much interest and speculation.

Early in July an enthusiastic neighbour had phoned a newspaper and told them our story. A reporter was on the doorstep at once and a photographer came too.

'Can you manage to lift the wheelchair now?' he asked me.

'Of course I can lift it,' I replied indignantly. 'I'll even hold it up above my head if you like.' How I regretted that piece of showing off! The picture and article covered the front page and we were completely unprepared for the interest it aroused. Suddenly the phone never seemed to stop ringing. Reporters from other magazines and papers arrived and their inaccurate accounts of our personal life caused us terrible embarrassment. People stood outside our house trying to see in through the windows and when we walked down the street we were conscious of people in cars pointing us out to each other as they drove by. One lady spent most of a Saturday looking through the letter box, 'just to see her walking round the house'.

As a family we were all beginning to feel horribly exposed, and when the ITV news rang up, we felt it was all getting out of hand.

'No, thank you,' I said firmly, 'we would much prefer that you didn't come and film us.'

'But we show so much bad news,' he pointed out. 'Don't you want to share a bit of happiness for a change?' I felt mean, but after years of isolation inside my own house all this sudden attention was decidedly traumatic. 'This is the most beautiful thing which has ever happened to us,' I thought miserably. 'Why can't we be allowed to enjoy it in peace? The quicker we disappear back into the country the better.'

Then something happened at a wedding in Mayfield on July 15th. Grace's son was being married, and when she had first asked us, months before, Tony said we could only go to the service. Receptions and parties of any kind had really become impossible for me. The noise of people chattering, and the swirl of movement round my wheelchair used to make me so giddy. In early July we had to write to the bride's mother to ask if we could come to the buffet lunch after all.

It was such fun walking about the marquee with Tony and talking to anyone who looked interesting, instead of sitting in the corner hoping they might come over to me. Standing up holding a drink is such an ordinary thing most people never even think about it, but it made me feel positively emancipated. People really do treat you quite differently when you are standing up. Instead of having to let Tony go up to the buffet table and select what he imagined I might like (or what he thought would be good for me), I could chose my own food, and came away with a rather vulgar amount!

During the meal we were sitting at a table talking to a most interesting man. We seemed to have discussed everything under the sun when he suddenly said, 'Do you happen to believe in miracles and all that stuff?' Before we could answer he continued. 'There was some woman on the front page of the paper recently, holding her wheelchair up over her head. Do you think it was all a fake?'

'Well actually I happen to know it wasn't,' I began diffidently. 'You see I'm the woman.' If only I could have taken a photo of his face.

'I've had arthritis for years,' he said wistfully, 'but I never thought there was any hope.' We were still talking about healing when the bride and groom finally left.

That night we saw our dread of exposure in a completely new light. Perhaps the TV reporter was right. We had been given a very special gift. We could keep it for ourselves or decide to share the joy of it with other people. If it had not been for that man in the wedding marquee, I might not be writing this book now.

I first hit the most baffling and painful part of my new life just a very few days after Haslemere. I had been for a long

186

early morning walk in the country and was coming back along the lane where I had so often 'bugged' near Tony's allotment. A car was parked in the lay-by and a man was setting up a wheelchair. As I drew nearer he lifted his wife from the front seat and with great difficulty, deposited her in the chair.

'Oh, good,' I thought, 'someone else has discovered this is the best wheelchair run in the district.' I hurried forward to say hello, quite forgetting I was no longer in my Bug. Had I been we would have become friends in seconds with a thousand things in common. Instead she sat there looking up at me coldly as if she thought I had come to patronise her. After 'Good morning' there did not seem to be anything else to say. I wanted to tell her, 'I'm not really part of the "well world", I'm still one of *us*. I'm used to sitting in a chair too, you know.' But how could I possibly explain all that? She would have thought I was nutty.

'Have a nice . . . er . . . ride,' I said awkwardly and hurriedly turned away. I was crying. It was not pity, she would have hated that, it was just knowing what wheelchairs feel like.

The tears were also selfish. I was crying for a lost identity. Would my other close friends look at me coldly like that now? I had met some very special people during the last six years. Their maturity and courage in the face of adversity had inspired me. I had been proud to be one of them and counted by them as a friend. Once I had allowed myself to join their identity group I felt safe because I finally knew into which box I fitted. Now, the 'reverse adjustment' was being just as difficult.

'Where do I fit now?' I thought as I walked back towards town. It felt like being suspended in a state of limbo.

However, as I neared home I became aware of a deeper grief. The circle of friends who have a physical handicap now numbered hundreds, and they had been my support. In the same way I had been theirs. For the first time I began to ask myself how they were going to react to my sudden return to

187

health. Would they feel as I had done when I met Julie Sheldon? Suppose I disturbed their peace – made them feel God isn't fair?

Later in the morning I happened to glance at the calendar. 'July 3rd, 1.30   Brenda and Chris Baalham.' It was a date I had been eagerly anticipating for several months. Brenda (who has rheumatoid arthritis) and I had been corresponding for some years. Neither of us could use a pen so we were 'computer friends' instead. We shared an interest in writing and worked for the same magazines, but even though we seemed to know every detail about each other's lives this was going to be the first time we had ever met. 'I must warn her before she arrives here,' I thought. But how could I explain? I drafted numerous letters to Brenda that day and deleted them all from the computer memory. In the end I never wrote at all. I behaved like an ostrich as I tried to pretend the day was never going to happen.

But it did. I watched her husband Chris lift the wheelchair out of the car from my window. Her two little boys were just as I had imagined they would be. How will Brenda feel I wondered as they all came up the ramp at the side of the house.

'We were looking for Jen,' said Chris as I opened the door. My throat felt as if I had swallowed a whole hedgehog. Why hadn't I written?

'But I'm Jen,' I heard myself saying brightly, 'and guess what?'

I could see a whole range of reactions flitting across Brenda's face and I felt as if I had betrayed her. The more embarrassed I was, the more brash and banal my remarks became.

It would not have been so bad if there had been fewer people around. Several other visitors dropped in that day and with some of my family and all of hers we never had a chance to talk properly.

Her boys were playing on the floor with Richard's outgrown cars, when one of them whispered hoarsely to Brenda,

188

'Mum, could God do that for you too?' I had to hurry away and make myself busy over a fresh pot of tea. Why? I raged in the kitchen. Why me? Why not her? Why not all my friends? Why? Why? Why? If I thought I had earned my healing by some act of good behaviour, the discovery of some new method of prayer or the superior brand of my faith, then I would not have felt so confused by the whole thing. Yet I could list many of my friends who deserved and desired healing more than I did. The whole thing bewildered me. It still does.

'I seem to have a bit of a cold,' I said firmly when I returned to the lounge. Just as they were leaving we had one moment of privacy. Chris was busy packing the chair into the boot of the car and Brenda was already strapped in the front. I crouched down so my eyes were level with hers through the open window.

'I'm sorry,' I whispered.

'Why?' she answered gently and I could see the peace I had always admired so much was still intact and invincible.

'I feel so guilty,' I mumbled.

'But you shouldn't,' she replied gently. 'You help us to know that we could all get better when the right time comes.' After a pause she added, 'I've given up bothering to try and understand God, it's so much more relaxing just to trust him.'

Most of my friends reacted to my healing as Brenda did, but for months my own head buzzed with unanswerable questions and every time I caught sight of a wheelchair, I burst into tears. It was very hard to keep reminding myself of my father's irritating maxim, "The Good Lord knows what he's a-doin' of."

Perhaps this confusion was not really resolved until I went to Loughborough in October. I had been asked by a medical student to take part in a healing service he and other undergraduates were organising. At the end (while people were being prayed for at the front) a large burly man pushed his way up to me and grabbed me by the arm.

'Come and talk to my fare,' he said without preamble. I

189

was slightly puzzled until I noticed a white taxi-driver's disc pinned to his jacket.

His grip on my arm was relentless as he marched me right to the back of the hall towards a red-and-grey wheelchair so like my own had been.

'He's a spastic and blind as a bloody bat too,' boomed my guide, but when the young man in the chair looked up and smiled at me I could see there was nothing disabled about his spirit. I pulled a chair up close to him, in spite of the taxi-driver's efforts to edge his way in between us.

'So you are actually Dave Preston,' I said when the young man told me his name. I had heard of him through the magazine. 'You work for local radio, don't you?' I also knew he edited a tape magazine for people with visual handicaps, lived successfully on his own and was another computer enthusiast.

'That's right,' put in the taxi-driver. 'I take him all over the show, he's a bloody marvel he is!' It was fascinating to talk to someone with a mind as keen as Dave's but after a while we were interrupted by two students.

'Can we have a private word?' they said to me. 'Why don't you take that poor young man up to the front for healing?' asked one of them enthusiastically when we had retired to a safe distance. To me Dave was not a 'poor young man', he was an interesting person living a full and useful life. I was about to tell them so indignantly when Dave's voice made us all jump. We had forgotten his hearing is highly trained.

'If the time was right, I would know,' he said gently. 'And if the first thing I ever see is the face of God, then that's fine by me.'

It was not difficult to guess that the taxi-driver disapproved of me and what I had said in the service about my healing. He obviously wanted to tell me so and kept on edging his chair closer still.

'It's easy for you – getting better like that,' he managed at last. 'But I've known this chap for a long time now and I've never heard him complain yet. He goes on with all this God business even when he doesn't get better. In my book that's a far bigger bloody miracle than yours.'

'Yes,' I said quietly, 'I'm beginning to think you're right.'

One day in the summer my friend Grace came over from Mayfield to see me.

'What do you enjoy most about this new life then?' she asked, and I told her about my long solitary walks in lonely places.

'I'm looking for a large black dog to protect me,' I told her. 'Minty is getting on a bit now.' Grace told me about Brodie, a black labrador puppy who had been born just two days after I was healed. Grace's daughter Lois had rescued her from the threat of being put down. Brodie had been blind from birth and no one wanted a handicapped dog.

'Lois can't possibly keep her,' said Grace, 'she has to go to work.'

The thought of having a blind puppy appealed to the whole family.

'I wouldn't have wanted to be written off just because I had a handicap,' I said, and Tony added, 'She could protect you just as well as any other dog.'

So, in September, Brodie arrived. Minty became a very proud 'guide dog for the blind' and the ingenious way Brodie overcomes her disability is a constant source of delight to us all. No one would ever guess she was blind if they saw her chasing Richard round the park using her highly developed senses of smell and hearing. She also has a phenomenal memory and never bumps her nose on the same chair leg twice (unless someone is mean enough to move it).

She is now fully grown, a magnificent-looking dog and her head and the set of her ears are sheer perfection. Some people, however, turn away when they pass her in the park, and two have even said, 'You're being cruel keeping her alive. She ought to be put to sleep.' Why? Because her eyes don't work? Everything else is perfect and she is blissfully happy. Because her eyes do not look attractive? But I could list a thousand things about her appearance and personality which are beautiful.

Somehow she sums up all I feel about disablement – and life in general. Why do we focus so much attention on the one thing which is a problem and ignore all the other things which are fine?

Yesterday was March 13th, the anniversary of the day I first knew I was going to be well. I celebrated by taking both the dogs for a walk round Mayfield. Unfortunately Tony could not come too, but being alone gave me a chance to think.

I rambled about the old familiar places which I knew so well in my memory. Everything was just the same – every footpath, stile and hedgerow. The church on the hill still had its safe 'unchangeable' quality. But I realised we were different.

We have talked so much about selling up and moving out into the wilds of Dartmoor or the Lake District to recapture our dream. I made such a fuss about losing it, but now it could easily be ours again we both feel we no longer want it. The years since we left Mayfield have turned our values upside down. People really have become more important now than 'frosted branches'.

As I jumped over the ditch into Fir Toll Woods I remembered the time when I last came here to think, the night after I had the dream. How bare and dismal the woods had looked then. Now the birds were singing again and the bluebells were already looking like shiny green fingers pushing up through the layer of dead leaves. Everywhere I looked were those almost imperceptible stirrings which promise the coming of a new spring. As I looked back over the years since that morning in February 1982 I realised life has often felt very wintry and bleak but as a family we have learnt so much through it all that there can be no regrets.

When I met Sir Harry Secombe again after I was better, he asked me if I thought my illness had been some kind of a test. I told him I was sure God was not that cruel. He would have to be a sadist to plan something like that for me and the people I love. On the other hand when difficulties came – simply because we are human – He used them for good, once we gave Him the chance.

People often say, 'Has the novelty of being well worn off yet?' Will it ever? I wondered as I walked along the path with the dogs at my heels and smelled the rich fresh scent of the earth.

All the same, life is not a continuous state of euphoria and, as I have said, some things are difficult. I have come to realise now that easy circumstances do not ensure happiness any more than difficult circumstances preclude it. Happiness still comes in isolated 'flashes' at the most unexpected moments.

'It must be fantastic to be free at last!' said an enthusiastic lady who also walks her dogs in the park.

'Yes, it's marvellous,' I replied and then thought, 'But what is freedom?' In the 'well world' I have discovered many people who appear to be free of physical and financial restraints yet they are actually far more trapped then Brenda or Dave. It is bitterness, self-pity and resentment which are the iron bars that imprison us, not our diseased bodies or distressing circumstances. The spirit can soar freely above all kinds of apparent obstacles when these prison bars are removed.

Last summer I discovered a poem. At first I thought it expressed how I felt when I was healed. Now I see that it describes the experience outside the post office seven years before.

The Healing

After so long, so long
in my tight prison,
with my familiar shackles
heavy on head and heart;
after so long, so long,
suddenly I see the bars

193

with the eyes God gave me,
touch the chains
with the hand God made me,
and suddenly, suddenly
(oh but my heart flies out of the dream
like a singing bird!)
suddenly I am free.

Virginia Thesiger

As I walked along by the little stream under the beech trees I thought about that day last summer when so many things changed. What exactly *did* happen to me then?

Technically, to be classed as a miracle by the Medical Bureau at Lourdes, a recovery must be totally impossible medically or by any other natural means – such as the restoration of an amputated leg. Although doctors could offer no cure for my condition, it could have improved by itself, just as such things as cancer suddenly disappear for no apparent reason. Yet it had not done so even after eight years. In fact my condition was gradually deteriorating. The sudden and total recovery I experienced during that prayer is hard to understand, yet most people I meet seem to have their own explanations. There was the old man who walked up the road the other day and stood watching me gardening in my little front 'pocket hankie'. When he had looked me up and down for some time he said,

'Well, it just goes to show, anyone can get better if they want to badly enough.' Was it mind over matter?

Then there was the woman who rushed up behind me in the High Street and hugged me until I gasped for breath.

'What a special kind of person you must be to be given such a miracle,' she gushed, but if she had known the unworthy thoughts that were going on inside my head she would have been forced to revise her ideas! Was it a spiritual blessing I managed to attain?

A TV reporter who had never met me before my recovery, told his colleague I was definitely a phoney.

'Just faked her way through the eight years – kept everyone on a string.' He must have thought I had an exceptional gift for acting, considering how many doctors I had managed to deceive, not to mention my family for so many years. Was I the victim of a wrong diagnosis in the first place?

A little old lady who often used to stop and talk to me in the Bug stood watching me walk up the road with shopping bags in either hand. 'Well,' she said, 'it just shows, doesn't it, there's someone up there after all?' Was it an answer to prayer?

Two medical friends asked me, 'But how do you know this virus isn't just lying dormant and won't flare up again in a few years' time?' I am confident that it won't, but there is no way I could prove that scientifically. So was it just a sudden remission?

'The body has remarkable powers of recuperation,' an elderly doctor told me. 'Surprising things sometimes happen quite by coincidence.' Did I simply recover by chance?

Everyone is entitled to their own opinions. Personally, I believe Jesus Christ touched me that day. The central pivot of the Christian faith is the belief that He is God, therefore torture and death could not destroy Him. He lives on by His spirit today. If this is so, then He must still have the same power now as He had when He wore the body of a man. Naturally He would still touch people in all manner of ways – emotionally and mentally as well as physically, sometimes by using natural means or medical science and occasionally intervening *super*naturally.

Although I believe all this, I am left asking the question, 'If Christ still has the same power and compassion, then why don't some people recover when they are prayed for?' I do not understand that, nor do I know why He should have given *me* back my health. It was a gift I did not ask for, deserve or expect. Yet I know He has no favourites and I am no more special to Him than my friends still in wheelchairs.

When I first stayed at Burrswood I met Bishop Morris Maddocks, who advises the Archbishops of Canterbury and

York on the ministry of health and healing. He once defined Christian healing as: 'Jesus Christ meeting you at the point of your need.' During the last nine years there were moments when both Tony and I felt quite desperate. On each of those occasions we experienced exactly what Bishop Maddocks describes. Yet sometimes it was impossible to recognise what our needs actually were. When I fell in the muddy bog I thought I needed physical healing in order to change the difficult circumstances which were sucking me down. Perhaps Christ saw that I had a greater need for peace, and soon the difficulties lost their destructive power.

I may emerge from this experience with many questions, but of one thing I am sure. When we cry out to God in our extremity, He hears and He always does the best thing. To my mind the gift of peace which He gave me in the muddy bog was every bit as miraculous as the gift of health which He gave me later at three fifteen on the afternoon of June 13th, 1990.

APPENDIX

Wendy's Story

Wendy was born in South Africa in a coloured township of Johannesburg and one of the first things she remembers is her mother's funeral. She was only three. Everyone else was crying, but her own grief had gone a long way beyond tears.

All the neighbours came to drink tea and shake their heads sadly.

'Poor man,' they whispered. 'How's he ever going to cope with two little kids all on his own?'

But it was only a few days later that a new 'mummy' joined them in the double bed the whole family had to share. Everyone seemed pleased about the arrangement – except for Wendy. She hated Lizzy from the very beginning and the antagonism was mutual. She remembers her new stepmother shouting:

'You're too black – you're nothing but dirt!' She herself was almost fair enough to pass as a 'white' but Wendy's skin was darker than the rest of the family. So Lizzy frequently plunged the little girl into baths of painfully hot water and scrubbed her until she was bleeding. 'You're ugly!' she would shout. 'You'll never have a boyfriend. No one could ever love you.' Those cruel words were to have a profound effect on Wendy's future life.

It never seemed possible to please Lizzy, however hard Wendy tried. While their father was out, both little girls were made to do all the household chores and were frequently beaten. When he came home, Lizzy would keep on complaining about their 'bad behaviour' until he took off his belt and beat them again. So Wendy grew into a lonely, frightened child who was convinced she was ugly, stupid and totally unworthy of love.

As she moved into her teens she longed for her father to be proud of her, but she lacked the confidence to perform well at school. If only she could be more like Julia, the star of the class. Everyone wanted to be Julia's friend. She was beautiful in every way and Wendy worshipped her. The day Julia decided to share her desk was the proudest moment of Wendy's life – though why Julia should wish to sit next to her mystified her completely.

'You shouldn't always screw your hair up in that band,' said Julia one day when she actually asked Wendy round to her home. 'It could be so pretty if you brushed it out.'

'Pretty?' thought Wendy incredulously. 'Me?'

When Julia had finished experimenting with Wendy's hair and showing her how to move gracefully, she declared, 'You're not ugly at all now.' But nothing could convince Wendy, and when the boys began to follow her round the school she wondered why they were staring at her. Yet Julia's friendship gave her confidence and when the exam results were announced she had done brilliantly. She was quite as astonished as her teachers.

'You do realise, don't you, that your daughter is highly intelligent?' The head master had visited Wendy's father in his own home just before she was due to leave school. 'We feel she should go on to university.' There were so few places for coloured students that they had to be brilliant to qualify for such a chance, but Wendy's father looked uneasy. Was he wondering what Lizzy would say?

'I'm afraid I could never afford it,' he said awkwardly.

Wendy drifted from one boring job to the next, until her ability was recognised at last and she was sent to college to do a course on computer programming and data processing.

Wendy's world changed overnight. At last she was successful and popular. In the evenings she worked as a waitress at a five-star hotel and with her earnings she bought the kind of clothes and make-up she had only ever dreamed about before. Soon the boys were positively queuing up for her attention and Lizzy's predictions were proved wrong.

Out of a class of forty, with only eleven passes, Wendy came out top in her exams, and as her presentation ceremony approached she hoped it would be the proudest moment of her father's life. She invited the whole family to the ceremony and in a burst of extravagance bought herself and her sister beautiful dresses to wear for the occasion. When the great day came, however, Wendy found her dress would no longer fit. She realised to her horror that she must be pregnant. The glamorous job she had been anticipating so much was impossible now. Marriage was out of the question, too; the baby's father was a boy she scarcely knew and their times together had not even been particularly enjoyable.

When her parents finally realised the situation, the row was appalling.

'So much for your precious daughter and her brains!' sneered Lizzy. 'I always told you she was useless.'

Wendy was forced to live at home, with Lizzy treating her like a slave once more. But when Maxine was finally born she knew that at last there was one human being in the world who would love her unconditionally.

Life was tough, all the same: Wendy had to work long hours in order to pay rent for a room and Georgie, the child minder. Her desperate need for security meant that she drifted into many casual relationships which often seemed to end in rejection and more pain. Then, three years later, she discovered she was pregnant again. It was a terrible moment. Lizzy's imaginary face smirked at her and Maxine's future seemed to be in danger. She felt there was no way she could have this baby, but abortions were illegal in South Africa and very expensive in the back streets. She borrowed the money in the end from a boyfriend, but felt by doing so that she had sold him her body.

She was already five months pregnant the day she left Maxine with Georgie and walked the five miles to the home of a woman who had once been a nurse. Much later that day she walked back again – and the five miles felt more like five hundred. She was bleeding heavily by the time she reached Georgie's home and in such intense pain she collapsed on the grass outside the door. Georgie, who was a very religious woman, was horrified when Wendy told her what she had done.

'How could you?' she exclaimed. 'You murderer!' It was dark and late and Maxine was crying in the sitting room. She could hardly leave Wendy lying out there, obviously in labour.

'You'd better come in I suppose,' Georgie said grudgingly, 'but I don't want my family to know anything about this. You go into my bedroom and mind you keep quiet.'

The next few hours were perhaps the worst of Wendy's life. Alone, she gave birth to twins, both perfect babies the size of her hand, and as she lay alone in the dark she grieved over them.

After that there did not seem to be much point in doing anything really. She could not work because the thought of those tiny babies kept on haunting her. There was no one left in the world to whom she could turn: even Georgie refused to speak to her. Stuck at home alone all day, she became even more depressed and Maxine's constant demands for attention were almost more than she could stand. Their relationship became so difficult that Georgie took the little girl away to live in her own home permanently.

'Life just isn't fair,' thought Wendy. She had nothing left now; she was ugly and useless just as Lizzy has always said. The world was full of people who possessed so much – good looks, money and happiness. Why should they have all the advantages while she was left out, alone and miserable? As she sat there she made a deliberate decision to use her wits to pull herself out of the mess her life had become – whatever it might cost other people.

In the end she became extremely successful, and rose from being a typist in Barclays Bank to developing their infant computer system into a national network – an unheard-of responsibility for a coloured girl in South Africa. But her real satisfaction in life seemed to come from breaking up other people's relationships and destroying their happiness.

One day her computer system developed a fault. A British technician called Ian was sent in to repair it. Wendy knew she was going to marry him the moment he walked into her office.

It felt like the chance to start life all over again when they arrived in England and, with Maxine, they settled in Haslemere. But Wendy did not seem to be able to leave her past behind in South Africa as easily as she had hoped. In an odd way she still felt chained to Lizzy and controlled by her. The marriage was explosive from the very beginning. She was used to men coming and going rapidly in her life, but this was the first time she had ever been in love and she was haunted by the fear of losing Ian. Her obsessive jealousy and the bitterness which always seemed to drive her relentlessly was poisoning their relationship.

They hoped a baby might help and Ian was delighted when Wendy found she was pregnant again. He longed for a son who would play football and cricket, but Wendy struggled constantly with a feeling that she was not worthy of happiness. She could not forget those little twins and a further abortion she had also had. This new baby would be sure to die as her punishment. She also became obsessed by guilt as she remembered all the people she had hurt and the relationships she had destroyed. Sometimes she felt compelled to bath three or four times a day, but she never lost the feeling of being dirty and defiled.

'Why can't you just decide to be happy and leave the past behind?' shouted Ian once in the middle of a major row.

'I would if only I could!' Wendy screamed back at him. She felt that her life was falling to pieces around her and there was nothing she could do to control it.

Then one night a strange thing happened. She dreamed she looked right up into heaven and there smiling down at her was the face of Christ Himself. Everything in her desired to know Him and be loved by Him and suddenly she realised He made her feel clean and beautiful – just as she longed to be. Like a tired and frightened child she lifted up her arms to Him but He gently shook His head.

'No,' He said, 'you're not quite ready yet.' She did not feel rejected because she knew instinctively that she must wait for something important to happen first.

She fought hard not to wake from the dream, which was so beautiful, but when she finally sat up in bed she was overwhelmed by a terrible feeling of loss. Her mother had been a devout Roman Catholic and, during Wendy's first three years, had often told her about someone called 'Lord Jesus' who loved her. Now, thinking about Him only seemed to increase her sense of shame.

When Richard was born, strong and healthy, Ian was enormously proud, but Wendy's anxiety would not allow her to relax night or day. She had to keep on looking into the baby's cot to make sure he was still breathing. 'I'm in prison,' she thought miserably, 'locked in by my own fears.'

Wendy had always viewed her neighbours with great suspicion, so when the mother of one of Maxine's school friends asked her to coffee she began to refuse. Then she stopped as she realised the neighbours name was Julia – the same as the 'superstar' who had befriended her long ago at school.

There was something about the way Julia opened her front door and the concern on her face when she said, 'How are you?' that broke down Wendy's reserve. During the next few months their friendship became very important to Wendy, but then one day Julia suddenly said, 'Why don't you come to church with me this Sunday? Maxine would love it.' Wendy was staggered.

'Me? Go to church?' she laughed. 'I couldn't look God in the face!'

'Come on, just try it once,' pleaded Julie. Very reluctantly Wendy went, but she hated every minute of the service. 'I'll never come back here,' she vowed. But the next Sunday morning she found herself there once again.

'This is ridiculous,' she thought as she walked into church on the third Sunday running.

That day something was said in the sermon which made Wendy very angry. She felt the preacher was talking about her and her private past as if he knew everything about it. Yet how could he possibly do so? During the week she went round to his house in order to try and straighten out the whole affair.

He explained that he knew nothing whatsoever about her, but perhaps God wanted her to know that He loved her very specially.

'How could He?' said Wendy wistfully. 'Surely there are some things which can't ever be forgiven – we just have to take the punishment coming to us.'

Quietly he explained that God loved people so much He came down himself and lived in the body of Jesus. He allowed men to put Him to death so that He could take the punishment for anything she could ever have done wrong. Slowly Wendy began to realise that carrying her own guilt about with her was actually crippling her. If she handed it to Christ in exchange for His forgiveness she could be rid of it for ever.

'I'd like that,' she said wistfully.

As they prayed she felt certain that she was being freed from her past, and after a few days she realised she had also lost the feeling of being dirty. 'I felt white all the way through,' was how she described it. 'And after I prayed with Julia later I even lost my fear of losing the baby.'

All this had only quite recently happened when I asked Wendy to pray for me at three fifteen on the afternoon of Wednesday, June 13th. She knew she had received forgiveness, but still she felt it would take years of holy living before she could earn the right to be used by God.

'I did not realise then,' she said, 'that in God's eyes no one is second class.'

WHERE HAVE YOU GONE, GOD?

Jennifer Rees Larcombe

Every Christian goes through a period at some time in their life when their relationship with God becomes dull or painful. For some, it happens at times of great success; others find that difficulties with health, relationships or career cause them to feel that God has abandoned them. Many can find no apparent reason for the spiritual 'desert' they are in.

'When we believe God answers prayer miraculously, it makes the tragedies of life harder to accept,' says Jennifer Rees Larcombe. Before writing *Where Have You Gone, God?* she contacted over a thousand people who, at some time in their Christian lives, felt far from God. Their experience, and the wisdom of Christians down the ages, combine to make a book of comfort and hope. 'There are no easy answers,' says Jennifer Rees Larcombe. 'Spiritual deserts are terrible, but they pass and through them, our love for God is so often strengthened enormously.'

LEANING ON A SPIDER'S WEB

Jennifer Rees Larcombe

A Novel of drama and suspense to
the very last pages

The inhabitants of Laburnum Terrace are oblivious of the threat hanging over them. Living and loving, laughing and sometimes crying, they have built a world which seems comfortable and secure enough. But is it?

When the aircraft plunges from the sky at 5.00 a.m. one morning, the world of Laburnum Terrace is shattered to its core. The values on which the inhabitants have built their lives are put to the test, and some prove as fragile as spiders' webs.